A Gift in Wolf's Clothing

Life With Diabetes

RACHEL A. GIFFORD, RN, MN, CDE

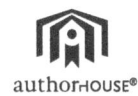

authorHOUSE®

AuthorHouse™
1663 Liberty Drive, Suite 200
Bloomington, IN 47403
www.authorhouse.com
Phone: 1-800-839-8640

First published by AuthorHouse 10/10/2007

ISBN: 978-1-4343-4333-8 (sc)

Library of Congress Control Number: 2007907714

Printed in the United States of America
Bloomington, Indiana

This book is printed on acid-free paper.

"Reading A Gift in Wolf's Clothing has made me a better doctor. Anyone who reads it will have a better understanding of what it is like to live with a chronic disease. In A Gift in Wolf's Clothing Rachel Gifford illustrates lessons diabetes has taught her by recounting childhood and adolescent interactions with parents, friends, and health care professionals. The vignettes are sometimes funny, often sad, and always poignant.
Charles Reasner M.D, Professor of Medicine and Medical Director of the Texas Diabetes Institute, University of Texas Health Sciences Center in San Antonio

"An engaging and insightful guide for anyone coping with diabetes, from someone in the trenches who shares invaluable lessons learned along the journey."
Patrick Perry Managing Editor, Saturday Evening Post

"In a world where difficulties often arrive as Visiting Instructors, A Gift in Wolf's Clothing hits the nail on the head. The humor is great, the pain is real, and the voice rings true."
Rev. Duke Tufty, Chairman of the Board, Unity

"With insight, humor, and pathos, Rachel Gifford has told a memorable story of diabetes."
James S. Hirsch, NY Times bestselling author, and author of "Cheating Destiny: Living with Diabetes, America's Biggest Epidemic"

"I urge all physicians and other providers of care for patients with diabetes to read this important book and to let it open their hearts and minds to the Wolf known as diabetes. I wish I had had this book to read when I was in my early years of medical practice. It would have helped me understand the thoughts, fears, and concerns of a young person with diabetes. It would have helped me prevent much mental and physical trauma in my patients, as well as in my own family, when my daughter discovered that she had Type 1 diabetes (at age 32) and my son-in-law when he was diagnosed three months later with Type 2 diabetes. We non-diabetic physicians cannot fully appreciate what it means to be a person who has diabetes. However, on reading about this first-hand struggle with day-to-day management of this disease, it makes things much clearer."
Royce Keilers, DO, FACOFP, Past President, ACOFP, Liaison AOA/ ACOFP/ADA
Father of a diabetic daughter and son-in-law

DEDICATION

For all of us who have diabetes. May we find our *voices* and use them to heal ourselves, change the healthcare system, and rock the world.

ACKNOWLEDGEMENTS

I'd like to express my deep appreciation to the first family I knew: The late Arthur Gifford, who taught me to be strong, tough, and always finish anything I started,

Nancy Gifford, who taught me to be spunky, and that having fun is essential to life,

Janis Gifford Day, who plowed the field of diabetes before I came aboard, and who is my life-long comrade with this devil disease, and Arthur Holland Gifford (Holly), who helped me know life changes – and – at the same time stays the same. We've all dealt with diabetes from our own personal window pane.

Thanking Randy Frazee, my husband, is a joy. His simple and unwavering belief in me made me realize I not only could write this book, but that thoughts otherwise simply were not compatible with life as he knew it. He is my Rock of Gibraltar.

Carol Newman was the first real-life-author I ever knew, and she generously shared her insights, expertise and wisdom. Had I not known her, this book would still be on my to-do list. Lawrence and Suella Walsh, superb authors of wonderful stories, have been my teachers, mentors and encouragers. In terms of Book Midwifery, these three folks have tended one of the longest births known to humankind.

I want to thank Lucy Sikes whose constant wisdom, compassion and prodding have helped me heal many wounds, uncover my heart's desires, and also keep moving toward them. She reminds me that magic is real and permeates the world. I am grateful to her for that immeasurable gift. Kathy Knapp gave my book its first informal edit, and encouraged me to keep going. Thank you, my friend. Then there are the "girls" from Carol Newman's Writing Group...holy cow! To name a few - Stephanie Hughes, Marilyn O'Hearne, Betty Swisher, Sue Monaghan, Jan Davis and Jane Rogers - always laughed at what I wanted laughed at, suggested improvements on stuff that needed improving, and overall reflected in their eyes that my story could help people, and make a positive difference in the world. Thank you, *thank you*. Thank. You.

FORWARD

When I agreed to review and comment on *A Gift in Wolf's Clothing: Life with Diabetes*, for Rachel, my long-time and dear friend, little did I realize what a moving experience reading this book would be. This is a girls' coming of age story that Judy Blume would be proud to have written. It is a book that all of us associated with diabetes should read and learn from. In my thirty-plus years of involvement in diabetes research, education and patient care, I have never before read such a compelling story of what it is like for a child to develop, adjust to and live with diabetes. I believe there are many similarities for adults who develop the disease as well. Nor have I read a book that so entertainingly, yet devastatingly points out the stupid and unfeeling things that health professionals do in the course of treating diabetes. If you are or have a child with diabetes, if you care for people with diabetes or if you are training to become someone who will care for children or adults with diabetes, buy this book and take its lessons to heart. Thanks Rachel for sharing your story with us.

Charles M. Clark Jr., M.D.
Associate Dean, Continuing Medical Education
Professor of Medicine & Pharmacology
Indiana University School of Medicine

INTRODUCTION

My greatest hope for this book is that it will change your life. For the better. We all get huffed-and-puffed by a Wolf or two, in our lives, and though I don't know *why* that is, I notice that it is. I've learned some amazing things from my Wolf called Diabetes. If I had learned those things in an easier way, that would have been fine with me, but that's not how it happened. Would I give up diabetes? In a heartbeat. Would I give up what I've learned from it? Not on your life – or mine.

A Gift in Wolf's Clothing isn't as clear a title as *10 Easy Ways to Fix Your Car*, so let me explain. Diabetes came to my door as the absolute worst Wolf I could imagine. Living with an older sister who had diabetes gave me a horror of the disease that you will understand better as you read the following chapters. In short, I watched my sister have seizures from low blood sugar, and run from our parents at insulin shot time. Because of diabetes, I saw her cry more tears than any kid should ever cry. I saw my parents' shoulders bend and nearly fold under the weight, but they never gave up. This Wolf had long shiny blood-stained fangs, and it waited close to the door to snag its prey. Wolf never left: twenty-four hours a day, seven days a week, for all the days of my sister's life. Because diabetes runs in families, I knew Wolf might be waiting for me as well. I was right. This part of my life is Section One – The Beginning of the End.

Those early days of Wolf terror were slowly replaced: hour by hour, day by day, learning by learning, over the years. I began to see the Gift under the fangs. From time to time, I saw a tender look in Wolf's huge yellow eyes...wanting to help me in a way that only shows up when I turned around to look behind me. When I glanced back at my trail, sometimes I saw Wolf prints with deep claws and evidence of a body being dragged behind. Other times I saw only Wolf prints. Where was I? As time went by, more often I saw Wolf and Rachel prints walking...hand in hand? This is Section Two: The End of The Beginning – Learning How to Think Like a Pancreas.

For nearly four decades Wolf and I have lived in the same body. Wolf is somewhat gray these days; often appearing friendlier. Yet there are days, and even more fearful nights, when Wolf rises with ferocity, flashing claws that once again threaten my life.

Wolf has taught me much; led me deep into the cause for why I am here, and pulled me down into the demons of my soul...only to shove me into reaching for courage to rise up again. Wolf has been my greatest enemy, and my stoutest teacher. We all have a Wolf; it just wears different clothes. Although we may befriend our Wolf, it cannot be domesticated. Wolf is a wild animal. You can only learn to live with an unspoken trust between the two of you. When the Call of the Wild rings through the frozen night air, you and Wolf will see fire rise in each others' eyes, and hopefully that fire is a passion that brings you together to make this world a better place. It's worth a try.

PROLOGUE

This happened after I had lived with diabetes for a year, and passed from sixth to seventh grade. Contrary to the doctors' warnings, I was still alive, had not gone blind, gotten kidney failure or had my legs amputated from gangrene. I had learned what gangrene was however, and the thought of it made me queasy.

I accepted the imperatives of diabetes: turning my pee funny colors four times a day *regardless* of where I was, having my insulin and syringe available for a shot before breakfast and supper (which I began to call dinner, like my friends...fitting in had become imperative, too), *always* carrying candy with me in case of low blood sugar, *always* thinking ahead by eating or packing a snack when I wanted to exercise, and so forth, and so on, ad nauseum. Life had become a long list of life-or-death-have-to-do's. The critical factor was: I had it mastered.

One week after my one year anniversary, my sister, Janis, and I had our diabetes check-up visit to the doctor. We were up early for the three hour drive from our home in Memphis, Missouri, to the Medical Center.

"You got everything?" Janis was doing the big-sister-thing, to make sure I was ready for the visit. This was funny, because despite her being three-and-a-half years older, usually she was the one who forgot stuff.

"Yep." I had packed insulin, syringes, alcohol wipes, snacks, urine tester, record sheets – both completed and blank - black, blue and red ink pens, pencils and crayons.

"Great! Let's go." She grinned and winked.

We both knew The Game would begin once we started our long trek to the doctor. The three hour drive to University Medical Center in Columbia, Missouri, took Dad about two hours and thirty minutes if

1

Mom was snoozing. Sometimes Janis and I completed our record sheets with urine test results, insulin taken, exercise, and other notations every day according to expectations of the god-doctors, like someone would in a perfect world. Other times we were less than perfect, so record sheets showed glaring blank spots. In the past few months, all my urine tests were negative, and my insulin dose had not changed. Writing that down bored me stiff, so I did not. Janis had had diabetes so long the whole thing bored her comatose, so she did what she needed for self-care without bothering to record the procedure. After all, one would expect a physician to know the procedure without our explaining it to him. One might be wrong.

Hence, The Game.

We devised beautifully completed record sheets in the car on the way to the clinic, and provided a creative impromptu performance in the doctor's office. Our methods were quite clever. We filled out record sheets with different colors of ink, and even interspersed a few entries in pencil or crayon. After all, one would not be expected to use the same writing utensil day after day for months at a time. Then we wadded up the corners, added a few tears, smudges and even stomped on some of them for antiquing. It had a good effect.

On the way out of town we made our usual stop at Granny's house for her home made lunch and snacks. Today she gave us steak sandwiches, fresh oranges and apples, sugar-free Jell-O with sugar-free fruit in it, and home made angel food cake. I had not accepted angel food cake as a substitute for chocolate cake, but it was still a treat having Granny make it for us; she made everything from scratch.

"Hon, you don't look like the same little girl I knew a year ago." Granny looked from me to my sixth-grade picture displayed on her coffee table. "You've grown up." She looked a little sad, but mostly puzzled.

I was relieved. I had changed irreparably since sixth grade; it was only right that it showed. "Love you, Granny...gotta go." We hugged, and I toted the lunch to the car.

The trip was uneventful, and finding our way to clinic was old hat by now. This would be an abbreviated version of our six month appointments, leaving out the physical exam and hopefully, the med students.

The nurse weighed and measured us, asked if we had been sick since our previous visit, and showed us our growth charts. "Janis, your weight is stable and you're a half inch taller than you were six months ago. Rachel, your weight is two pounds less than six months ago and you're two-and-a-half inches taller."

I was encouraged. Over the past year my height and weight had caught up with each other, putting me at the fiftieth percentile for both. I no longer shopped in the "Chubette" department. The day I bought my first dress at a normal store had been stupendous, and I actually had a waistline.

The nurse ushered Janis and me into the exam room (known to us as the Holding Tank), provided us with hospital gowns, and left our charts on the table. We exchanged glances. Sure...why not?

Janis opened her chart and read aloud what the nurse had written. "Seventeen-year-old post pubertal female presents to clinic for evaluation of diabetes. No complaints." She looked at me. "No complaints? How do they know? Nobody asked me." She picked up my chart and read. "Thirteen-year-old pubertal female presents to clinic for evaluation of diabetes. No complaints." She looked at me again. "Did they ask you for complaints?"

"Nope."

"Well, maybe we should give them some. You got any?"

"Yeah, this hospital gown is pretty trashy. And I'm tired of waiting for the doctor."

Janis wrote in my chart. "Any other complaints you want me to put in here?"

I thought for a few moments. "Yeah. Put down they need to get more chairs in these rooms. I'm tired of sitting on this stupid exam table. Why do you always get the chair, anyway?"

"I'm older. More chairs..." She wrote in the chart. "Okay, d'zat do it?"

"That's enough for now."

"Now for my complaints. I don't want to see any med students this time. They're *beyond* goofy." She picked up her chart and wrote several sentences, then read aloud, "Medical students are complainable, and I prefer not to see any at this visit."

"Good! Did you sign your name? I think you're supposed to sign anything you write in the chart."

"Yep. Janis L. Gifford – Post pubertal Complainer." We broke into giggles.

"You girls sound like you're having fun in here." Dr. Jackson walked in, followed by three medical students who – for the life of me – triggered an instant image of Larry, Curly and Moe.

Janis and I tried to sober, but it was not easy.

"Do you have your record sheets?"

I handed him mine, and Janis pulled hers from her purse. We exchanged glances and stifled our snickers.

Dr. Jackson looked over the records. "Looks good. You girls are really compliant."

I heard Janis sputter. For us the word "compliant" gave the crawly feeling of a tick on your neck. It was a ridiculous term that meant blindly following whatever the god-doctor said without so much as one calculated, independent thought. We knew it was impossible for anyone, who did not live everyday with diabetes, to have an inkling of how much thinking, planning, willpower, and sheer effort it required just to get out the door in the morning – *every* morning. We had great self-respect in doing what it took to keep ourselves healthy. "Compliance" was a blatant insult.

Janis was better at this than me. "Yeah, it takes a lot of work, you know." She left it at that; I was surprised.

Dr. Jackson looked at her. "Yes, I'm sure it does." He opened her medical chart. There was a pregnant pause until he read, "Complainable, eh? Hm....Janis, are you aware the chart is a legal document?" He gave her a stern look over the top of his glasses.

Janis swallowed. "Whose legal document is it? I see my name printed on the outside." She was a master.

"Well, yes, it does have your name on the outside. However, it's not for trivial journalism."

Janis stood to her full height of five-feet-eight-inches and looked eye-to-eye with Dr. Jackson. "I'd like you to know, I'm not a trivial journalist! The nurse wrote that I had no complaints, and I can tell you that's a falsehood. If the chart is a legal document, it needs to contain the truth." Her eyes snapped...it was scary.

Dr. Jackson sighed and laid the chart back on the table. "So, how is school going, Janis?"

"Fine, thanks. How is school for you guys?" Janis changed roles, smiling toward the Three Stooges who suddenly snapped to attention, but were obviously at a complete loss for words.

"Okay..." Dr. Jackson moved his conversation away from Janis. He picked up my chart and began to read. The room was silent. "So...we have trashy hospital gowns and need more chairs?" He turned to one of the med students. "Frank, would you go get another chair for Miss Gifford?"

Frank (who in my mind was Curly) looked bewildered, but nodded quickly and left the room.

Dr. Jackson turned to Moe and went into professor mode. "Can you give us an overview of appropriate education for the child with diabetes?"

Moe cocked his head, his eyes glazed over, and lo, he spake, quoting from the stone tablets in his mind: *"Verily, I say unto you, he who hath diabetes shall suffer all the days of his life. The light of his eyes shall grow dim, and he shall see neither by the light of day, nor the stars of night. His kidneys shall fail him, and the days of his life will be sustained on the dialysis machine. He who has diabetes shalt not go bare-footed, as wounds upon his feet shall not heal, but rather fester into gangrene, and cause ripping and tearing of the limb from his body. Yay, I say unto you, woe be unto that diabetic who doth not harken and hold fast unto every word that uttereth from the mouths of god-doctors, as that one shall surely die."*

That may not be verbatim.

Dr. Jackson nodded and turned to Janis and me, who sat dazed from Moe's herald of doom. "Girls, you have a hell of a disease."

Janis squinted at him when he said, "...hell...", because grown-ups weren't supposed to say that in front of kids.

"And," he continued, "it can kill you – or - you can manage it. You have to think more, plan more, and be smarter than anyone else around you." He paused, and a gentle grin lurked behind his doctor veneer, "It's okay though, because I know you can do it."

Just then Curly burst in with a chair. I hopped off the exam table and sat down.

Janis nodded toward Moe. "Thanks for the recitation." Then she turned toward Dr. Jackson. "And thanks for the words of wisdom, Dr. J. Look forward to seeing you next visit." Janis saluted, and with that they were dismissed.

Lessons Learned:
1. I am not, nor will I ever be, compliant.
2. Janis is not a trivial journalist, and some day she might be a famous actress.
3. In the past twelve months I have shed the skin of childhood. Though it ripped me raw, I am grateful to be done with it.
4. Medical authority figures of the world can be managed; it just takes experience and backbone.

Part One – The Beginning of the End

CHAPTER 1

You might be wondering about how life was before I got diabetes. Well, as a little kid my life had its ups and downs. My earliest fears of diabetes came from watching my older sister, Janis, who had developed the disease when she was only one-and-one-half; two years before I was born. Whenever I felt sad, I remembered two things. The first one I learned in church - God is always there and loves me, and the second one I learned from Mom – I am very lucky, because I don't have to take shots for the rest of my life. That reality worked for quite a few years; then I got diabetes. It wiped out the second premise, and made the first one pretty shaky.

I'm a thinking person. That's not always so good. "You think too much, Rachel!" Granny would say. It didn't change me, though. Mom and Dad both taught school, and we had a farm, too, but I think it was the teacher in them that recited the symptoms of diabetes to my brother, Holly – or Arthur Holland Gifford, when Mom was really mad – and me, since, well...forever. Even though Holly was two years younger than me, just a kid of ten-years-old, they wanted to be sure we both knew what to look for in case we got it.

> Symptom No. 1 – Very thirsty
> Symptom No. 2 – Going to the bathroom a lot
> Symptom No. 3 – Very hungry
> Symptom No. 4 – Feeling really tired or sleepy
> Symptom No. 5 – An illness or sore that would not heal.

I had those symptoms memorized, and could recite them in my sleep. It was Number 5 that weighed on my mind when my twelfth birthday rolled around on February twelfth, same as Abraham Lincoln's, only more recent. I had a sore throat going on two weeks, and felt sick all over, not just in my throat. Even Mom and Dad didn't know how bad I felt.

Mom said I should stay home from school and rest. She taught first grade, and had promised that when her class went out for recess she would call to check on me. I slept until about ten-thirty a.m. By eleven a.m., I was worn out with resting, and started thinking. I wondered if I had diabetes. It may seem to you like a big jump to go from feeling sick to wondering about diabetes, but that's because you didn't grow up in a house where diabetes permeated every cell and pore of life. If you had, and you were a thinker, quick as a wink you would be there, too.

Janis had a urine tester kit that she used to check her diabetes control three or four times a day. It was really cool, with a test tube, an eye dropper for putting water and urine in the test tube, a pill to put in the test tube, and one you put under the test tube. Then you set that pill on fire, to make the concoction in the test tube boil. It was indubitably cool. Indubitably is a thinker's word. It means you've thought on something from every conceivable angle, and come to a final and irrefutable conclusion.

I wandered into the bathroom, figuring the test would be an interesting way to kill time. I peed in the cup and put drops of pee and water in the test tube. I dropped in the blue pill, and set the little white pill on fire under the test tube. I'm not a pyromaniac, but I did enjoy seeing the mixture boil and turn colors. Blue meant there was no sugar and everything was good, green meant some sugar, and bright red was something you never wanted to see.

My test turned blue. But as it boiled longer it turned green. Then it turned orange-red...like a Smokey-the-Bear-forest-fire. I held my breath, and blinked hard. Maybe I didn't clean the test tube well enough before I started. Yes, that had to be it!

I dumped the orange stuff, and scrubbed the test tube within an inch of its glassy life. Deep breath in, out, in, out. Meticulously, I repeated each step. I lit the white pill, and the mixture began to boil. As I watched, my mind wandered to all that I knew about diabetes.

~~~~~~

Janis had to take three shots every day of her life. She would have to, every day, forever. She often cried, and ran away from Mom and Dad at shot time. A lot of times, she had seizures at night because her blood sugar dropped while she slept. It was my job to listen for her to breathe funny or for her bed to squeak. Those were the signs for me to alert Mom or Dad. I really tried to pay attention, but sometimes I slept too soundly, and woke up to a free-for-all in our bedroom.

Janis would lay on her bed writhing, screaming and crying. Dad would pin her down and yell, while Mom wheedled and coaxed Janis, trying to pour Karo syrup or orange juice in her mouth. It was a spectacle that made me think of the Reign of Terror during the French Revolution that my history book talked about. The book said, *"Peasants did not know when or where death would strike next."*

Often Janis slapped the orange juice or syrup from Mom's hand. It flew across the room as Janis blindly seized. Finally, she lay motionless. The scene quieted as the Reign of Terror slinked underground. Mom and I would mop up sticky syrup, speaking only if required, and then in hushed tones. Mom would be pale. Dad would look like he had wrestled a demon. Then we would try to sleep. But I had to keep listening for that bed squeak.

The morning-after Janis remembered nothing, but try as I might, I could not forget. The scene was etched in my mind like names on a tombstone.

Janis would have a throbbing headache, and sometimes got nauseated and threw up. Mom usually called Granny to come stay with Janis while the rest of us went to school. You can't send someone to school sick. It's inhumane.

I thought one night she might not come out of the seizure. Or she might choke on the syrup, and I wouldn't have a sister anymore. Mom and Dad thought so, too. I saw the fear gnaw their insides. They never talked about it in front of us three kids, but I knew it was there. In a way it glued them together.

~~~~~~

I looked back at the test tube. The mixture had finished boiling and it was bright, flaming orange. I ran blindly to the phone and dialed the principal's office at Mom's school. "This is Rachel Gifford. I have to talk to my mother immediately. This is a life-threatening emergency."

I heard a pause on the other end as Mrs. Milton, the secretary, caught her breath. "Honey, are you all right?"

"I. Need. My. Mother."

"I'll be right back."

The receiver thumped on the desk, and Mrs. Milton's chair grated across the floor. Her footsteps clicked loudly, then faded.

I waited. Tears dripped on the receiver. Mine? Was I crying? That had to stop; I couldn't blubber into the phone like a child. I bit my lip hard. Then I remembered people with diabetes don't heal like "normal" people, so I stopped.

"Rachel, are you okay?" Mom's voice sounded shaky.

"*MOM!!!* I have diabetes!! Oh no, oh no, oh noooo..." I was shrieking into the phone.

"What? Honey, what's wrong? What are you doing?"

"Oh, Mom...it's all over. I have diabetes. I tested my urine with Janis' kit, and its flaming red! What will I dooooo?" Sobs shook me so hard I dropped the phone. Between sobs I came up for air and retrieved it.

Mom came up for air about the same time. "Listen, I know you did the test for sugar, but that doesn't mean *for sure* you have diabetes. When I get home, we'll test your urine for ketones. That'll tell us more. I'll call Granny, and she can come stay with you. It's okay. Go back to bed or watch TV until I get home. Really, you're fine."

She sounded calm. It was reassuring, but deep in my heart I knew she was crying, too. She wouldn't let me know it, but in my mind I could see her face. Tears streamed down her cheeks and fell onto her favorite purple dress.

"Don't worry about me, Mom. I'll be okay. You can go back to class now." I tried to sound as calm as she had. I mostly succeeded, but I knew she saw my face in her mind, just as I'd seen hers.

Mom told me once that when Janis got diabetes, she and Dad had thought long and hard before having more children, for fear they might develop diabetes, too. She said the doctors reassured, saying it was unlikely; not to worry. You would think the doctors would know. You would be wrong.

Might I have been better off never being born?

I stumbled back to the bathroom and collapsed onto the toilet lid. I prayed a silent desperate prayer. *Dear God, please don't let me have diabetes. Please. Amen.* My brain spun into a tornado. That happens to thinkers. If I checked my urine for ketones I would know for sure if I had diabetes. Ketones meant your body had started to digest its own fat for nourishment, and it happened if you had diabetes. If I did not have ketones, I would have escaped the jaws of death. However, if I *did* have ketones... I had to do the test.

Ketones were measured in "none, small, moderate or large." Not at all precise, but the message gets through. My test showed "moderate". I lay down on the floor and cried until no more tears came out. Life as I knew it was over.

Lessons Learned:

1. Diabetes may be worse than death.
2. When people say, "The thing you fear most will never happen," they are wrong.

CHAPTER 2

In the hours and days that followed, details circled around me like piranhas. I called Mom back and told her the ketone news in a headed-for-the-firing-squad voice. Granny came. Mom and Dad called Dr. Jackson, Janis' diabetes doctor, who said to come to the Medical Center hospital on Monday. Today was Friday. Why was it okay with God for me to have diabetes? The words to "Jesus Loves Me" ran through my brain. Oh yeah?

It was decided Dad and I would go to the Medical Center hospital in Columbia, Missouri, which was three hours from home – might as well have been Siberia. Mom would stay home with Janis and Holly. The doctor said I would be there for two to three weeks. To a twelve-year-old, that is one, two-hundred-eighths of your life - basically an eternity.

Dad took me to school to get my books, so I could attend the hospital school, and keep up with my studies. Books and studies seemed irrelevant, but the notion brought a glimmer of hope. They represented routine and familiarity.

I packed the "Chubbette" dresses Mom and I had gotten in Ottumwa, Iowa. We had to go to a special store, known to my siblings as the Fat Store, to find my size. Mom had gotten me five dresses, two pairs of slacks and a cool blue blouse with windowpane check and a Peter Pan collar at the beginning of the school year. I knew she worried that I was overweight, probably because she hated being overweight herself, so she tried her best to help me look cute. I was grateful for her concern. And for the new clothes.

Monday morning came: The Trip to the End. Dad and I started early, before daylight. It was appropriate to travel the Trip to the End in pitch darkness. After driving a couple of hours we were hungry, so Dad stopped at a restaurant. Eating out as a pair, just Dad and me, was a huge treat. We were special to each other. Mom had so much to do taking care of Janis, that when I came along she kind of gave me to Dad. It was only fair. If Janis had the Disease, it was right she got the Mom. But now I had the Disease, too. I did not think Mom would change horses in mid-stream.

"Eat whatever you want, kiddo. This'll be your last chance." Dad gave me an ornery smile, as if we were conspiring to beat the devil at his own game.

I thought of my Chubbette dresses and paused. Then I ordered eggs, sausage, pancakes, coffee with cream and sugar, tomato juice, chocolate milk, a cinnamon roll, muffin, strawberries, and fresh biscuits. I was on death row, ordering my last meal.

Daddy smiled. Usually he curtailed restaurant orders to keep down the cost, but today he let me order it all. Even the coffee. Having coffee with Dad was a very big deal. I felt sick thinking of what lay ahead, but knowing Dad was with me made it easier. After all, *nobody* messed with Dad. He was tough. And he wasn't scared of anything in the world. He never had to tell me that; he wore it like a suit of armor. Even when he'd had his two heart attacks he wasn't scared. I think.

I tried to eat everything I ordered as that was the family rule, but it was too much. Dad and Mom were very serious about not ordering more than you could eat. It would waste food that might otherwise magically feed starving children in third world countries. Or even worse, in Dad's mind, it wasted money, which was always scarce.

"Don't worry, hon." Dad looked at me. "It's okay this time."

A reprieve; who cares if a man sins on his deathbed?

Then we got There - all too soon. I had managed a courageous front until we drove into the huge hospital complex. Once we were overshadowed by the tall gray buildings, tears fell out and dripped silently down my chin.

Daddy looked at me; I thought he might cry, too. "Hon, if there was any way I could take this for you, I would. But I can't."

I knew he meant it. Both parts.

Awful is a pale description of our experience. There must be better words: Hideous? Wretched? No, not big enough. I imagined the right word: Gargantuhorrificulous? Omnihellipresent? Sometimes even thinkers get stuck.

The hospital was huge, and we could not find the right floor. When we finally got there, the White Coat told me to take off all my clothes and put on a gown with no back in it. I remembered a World War II movie where Nazis told prisoners the same thing. Then the prisoners were sent to the gas chambers.

Next, White Coat wanted to draw blood. The man stuck me four times, probed the needle around, shoved it back and forth in my arm, all to no avail. I had bruises the size of oranges on both arms, and this idiot still rammed the needle around inside my skin. Dad clenched and unclenched his fists.

"Your veins seem to roll around. They're hard to hit." This came from White Coat, who I found out later was a medical student; not even a real doctor. I did not think he would be all that hard to hit. If I snatched my arm away I could land a smashing blow to his nose before he could blink twice. I would follow that with several swift kicks and maybe a body-slam. It was a comforting picture.

To this twelve-year-old thinker, the man epitomized not only a torturer, but incompetence, insensitivity and stupidity as well. On top of that he stunk. Had he fallen into a vat of alcohol or did he just use it for aftershave?

He told me matter-of-factly that they would "order labs" for every morning until my blood sugar stabilized. I sucked in my beath. Daddy was staying with a college friend in Columbia, so this meant that every morning, before Daddy even got to the hospital to help me and be by my side, these people (not an accurate word...Zombies? Aliens? Vampires?) would come for me with needles. And they would keep sticking until they got what they wanted. I needed to be dead. Rationally, there was no other choice.

Then came "physical examinations." I wondered how one would be graded on these exams. Being a Chubbette probably wouldn't get me very good scores. They were beyond intrusive, stripping away more layers of dignity and humanity. As they worked they took particular interest in informing me of my fate as a *diabetic.* I no longer had a Self, I had a label.

As a *Diabetic,* I must never again go bare-footed. I could get a cut that would never heal, and have to have my leg cut off. What would spring be like without running bare-foot through soft new grass? Apparently I would find out.

As a *Diabetic,* I must be aware that I could easily go blind, if I didn't follow my diet and obey all doctors' orders. This statement was accompanied by a long finger jabbing a staccato in my face to the words "blind", "obey", and "orders".

As a *Diabetic,* my kidneys might fail. If that happened, I would go on a kidney machine, but ultimately kidney failure would kill me.

As a *Diabetic,* it was likely I would die of a heart attack or stroke. I listened in a nightmare where ghouls and goblins discussed what to do to me, as I hung tied and dangling upside down from a tree limb. The next step could be putting me into a pot of boiling oil.

But it was not. The next step assigned me to a hospital room where I was told to get in bed. *What?* It was the middle of the day, and the sun was still up. But I got in and pulled the covers up to my eyes. I would have pulled them over my face, but I needed to keep an eye on things. White Coat left. I began to feel safer. Silly me. Another parade of doctors, medical students, and god-only-knows-who filed through, all of them wanted to poke, prod, and examine me. I was the resident exhibit.

The group Leaders took particular interest in announcing to their followers, "She's twelve years old, starting puberty. Diabetes may impede that. And as you can see, she's very fat."

Fat! Always fat. *I* knew I was fat. Anybody looking at me could *see* I was fat. Couldn't they just be quiet about it? NOOOOO! They undressed me, uncovered me, stared at me, and then announced in front of an entire group, "She's FAT!" Inside I cried. I screamed. I kicked them in the face. But outside...outside, I wouldn't let them see me cry. I went to a world where I could think and not feel.

So, I thought about the word impede. I had heard that word, but couldn't come up with the meaning. I tried to figure it out. The prefix "im" means not, like improper is not proper. "Ped"...could mean feet like in pedestrian or pedal, or it could mean children like in pediatrician. So impede could mean no feet or no children. Were they saying my puberty (I knew what that was, Mom told me) could be without feet? Without feet it couldn't go anywhere, so would it stop? I would never go into puberty? I'd never be a woman?

Or maybe I would be without children. Would diabetes keep me from ever having children?

Who were these freaks of nature? Who gave these Leaders permission to invade and humiliate me to their group of imprinting ducklings? When the fourth male White Coat came in (odd there were no women; had they killed them all?), and said the ubiquitous, "I'm Dr. Somebody, and I need to examine you," I told him it had already been done three times and he could go ask one of the other guys what they found.

He straightened himself up very tall, took on a grand air of authority, and said he *must* examine me. I wilted. It is hard to be tough when you're little, fat, female and outnumbered. Of all the things they stole, I missed my voice the most.

Finally Dr. Jackson, my *own* doctor, came in, followed by his own entourage of waddling, quacking White Coats. He looked at my eyes, which none of the others had seemed to notice, and his eyes softened. I had been crying. The truth was I couldn't stop crying. As forcefully as I walled up the pain, it continued to leak out. He asked the little White Coats to step outside.

Like a wounded animal, I implored him for mercy. "Dr. Jackson, they say I have to have blood drawn every morning until my blood sugar stabilizes. How long will that take? How long, Dr. Jackson? How many days? How long do I have to be here?"

Dr. Jackson was a short balding man with a round tummy. He often talked about his children, six girls and one boy. He looked down at me, perched precariously on the edge of the bed. He must have wondered if I was about to fall off.

"It might be only until tomorrow. We'll take it a day at a time. When your urine sugars are negative there won't be a need for the venipunctures... the blood tests."

Venipuncture, interesting word. The puncture part was right. I heard "...only tomorrow...," and grasped, almost visibly, at that hope. I felt like I needed to grab it with both hands and pull it in to protect my heart. "Dr. Jackson, I need to put my clothes on."

He softened again. His eyes looked like a daddy instead of a doctor. "After I leave, go in the bathroom, lock the door and get dressed. That way no one will accidentally walk in on you while you're changing."

Accidentally? These people believed they had the right, if not the responsibility, of slamming into my life as if they were headed for Normandy Beach. My tears stopped. "I will Dr. Jackson. Will you be back to see me later today?"

"I'll try." He walked quietly out of the room, softly closing the door behind him.

He didn't make it back. I locked myself in the bathroom and put on my clothes. I decided I would get dressed the next morning before the blood people came, to boost my courage for the occasion. I opened the bathroom door and walked, now as a human being, over to the window. From the eighth floor I looked out at rain and sleet pelting the cars in the street below. I rested my hot cheek against the cool glass.

One fast jump, that's all it would take. Yank the window up, dive out, feel the breeze as I flew down, and wake up in heaven. No more diabetes. No more doctors. No more venipunctures. Relief swept over me. I gripped the window handles, smooth and cool in my hands. Slowly, I inched the window up, focusing on the street below. I pushed my shoulder into the opening. Not wide enough. I shoved it up another foot. That would do.

Then Reality blared an argument. *"Oh yeah, right, Rachel. You jump out of here, and with your luck, you won't die. You'll live the rest of your life as a diabetic in a wheelchair. How does THAT sound?"*

Not good. I left the window where it was, and felt cold air whip across my chest. I thought of Daddy. My "daddy" who rescued me when I was afraid, became "Dad" when I was confident. Daddy had suffered two heart attacks, we'd almost lost him both times. I imagined him looking from the window, seeing me splattered across the street. Tears ran down his face. What if it made his heart attack again?

I had never seen Daddy cry. I could plunge to my own death, but could I drag him with me?

Lessons Learned:
1. Daddy couldn't always rescue me.
2. White Coats believe making me afraid of my disease is a smart thing to do. That is really weird.
3. A *diabetic* is no longer a human being.
4. White Coats think the title "doctor" is more important than the title "human". They are wrong.
5. Venipuncture is a painful, but legal form of torture.
6. In the hospital, having a bathroom door that locks is a good thing.

CHAPTER 3

Nighttime came, and so did Daddy. Visiting hours let him be with me for only one hour in the morning and two hours in the evening. I did not understand visiting hours. To get well, what could I possibly need more than Daddy? Were they locking him out, or me in? Either way smacked of poor judgment.

I heard his steps in the hallway, and my heart pounded. Then I heard his voice - Daddy was a bass, for sure. When he sang it was usually off-key, but the depth of his tone was unmistakable. I heard him laugh and greet someone. Could there be a more wonderful sound than Daddy's laugh? It came out like a bellow and filled whatever space it entered. Tears of relief streamed down my face. He was getting nearer, I could smell his cologne. Daddy wore Old Spice or English Leather. That's what Mom liked, so that's what he wore. It was simple. The door opened.

"Sweetheart...?"

I sat in the dark. The only streaks of light came from the window, which now was closed as tightly as I could get it. I choked back tears, but sobs took my throat.

He walked to the bed and sat beside me. His strong arms embraced me, arms that tossed bales of hay like I would toss a pillow, arms that engulfed me. Daddy's smell was that of a man who knew and loved physical activity. He could never be quiet for long, either vocally or physically. He was sweating. I imagined he spent much of his time away, walking. The smell of him brought comfort to my jangled nerves. I slumped against him, and sobbed until his shirt was soaked.

"It's okay." He wiped my tears with his big rough hands.

"Daddy, I was so scared. Please can you stay tonight? Please, Daddy? Dr. Jackson said they'd draw blood in the morning, and I can't do it by myself. I know I can't! Please?"

"We'll see, honey. We'll see." He held me close, and his heart next to mine thumped a rhythm of comfort. His courage flowed into me, but it wasn't enough.

"What did you have for supper?"

I cleared my throat. "No supper yet. They have to teach me to give myself a shot first, and then I can eat." Tears started again. I closed my eyes and sobs shook me.

His arms came back, and his soggy shirt pressed against my cheek.

The sobs faded more quickly this time.

"I'll go with you. We can do it together."

His words echoed through my head. "You can't. They said parents aren't allowed in the shot room."

"That doesn't apply to me. Where is this shot room?"

"I don't know, but we can ask a nurse."

He wiped my face with his handkerchief, took my hand, and led me into the hall as if we owned the world. A nurse came toward us wearing a nametag that said *Lonnie*.

"Excuse me, Lonnie. My daughter, Rachel, and I need to go to the shot room so she can take her first insulin injection. Would you help us?"

Lonnie looked at Dad, then down at me.

With all my crying, my eyes and nose must be red and swollen; I must look like a total disaster.

"Who are you, sir?"

"I'm Mr. Gifford, and this is my daughter, Rachel. She's quite hungry." Dad's voice sounded calm. He was not asking for assistance, he was letting it be known he expected it.

"Certainly, Mr. Gifford." Lonnie gave me a smile. She was pretty. Very tall and slender with short, thick black hair that was really cute. Her smile was friendly. She looked like she wasn't in a hospital at all, and talking with her made me feel like we were at the grocery store asking for the green bean aisle.

Lonnie led us down the hall, past the nurse's station, and we turned left into a little room that smelled overwhelmingly antiseptic. She checked a notebook with writing all over the pages, and said, "Okay, five and five."

It sounded mysterious to me, but there was little that had not been weird since I got to this place.

She pulled two glass vials from the refrigerator and laid a syringe on the counter. My face went numb.

Lonnie seemed to notice. She knelt down and looked into my eyes. Her eyes were brown like mine. I liked that.

"You can draw up your insulin tonight, but I'll help you with the injection. Is that okay with you?"

A grin tugged the corner of my mouth. "Um...okay.

"Hold the syringe like this. Then wipe off the bottle with alcohol..." Her voice trailed on, and apparently I did what she asked. However there wasn't much I remembered until after the shot, when she hugged me.

"You did great, Rachel! You're going to be a champ at this. You know, we'll have you teach other people how to do it!"

"Th....thank you, Lonnie."

She hugged me again. "I'll bring your dinner in a few minutes."

Sweet relief. Suddenly I remembered Dad; where was he? I caught a movement from the corner of my eye.

"You did *so* good, honey. You'll have this thing whipped in no time."

Was there a catch in his voice? He held me tightly. The spot where my tears had soaked his shirt was only a little damp now. He took my hand, and we walked back to the room. The halls didn't look as dark and scary. A light had crept in.

"Want to call Mom, hon?"

I had finished supper, and we both knew it was time to get out of this claustrophobic hospital room. I wasn't sure I wanted to talk with Mom, though. What if I cried again? I hated crying! It made my head hurt, my eyes hurt, my stomach hurt, and my nose run. It's all I had done since I got here.

"I...I don't know." We walked into the hall, and the antiseptic smell hit me. As we approached the phone I felt jumpy inside. "You talk first, okay?"

"Okay." He placed the call and I heard him speak to Mom. Tears burned in my eyes. I pinched myself and tried to remember to breathe. In, out. In, out. Slow, easy.

"Want to talk to Mom?"

I took deep breaths and shook my head no.

He handed me the phone anyway.

"Hu...." I cleared my throat. "Hullo, Maa...Mom." The tears were unstoppable. I covered my mouth and gave Daddy the phone. It was impossible. Damn! Why couldn't I stop crying? I was so out of control. I sat down and laid my face in my hands. After thinking "damn" it felt silly asking God for help, but who else was there? *God, please help me. When will this be over?*

"Ready to go somewhere else?" Daddy stood beside me, looking as though everything was okay. I wished this made me feel better, but it didn't. I couldn't rally.

As we walked to the cafeteria our steps echoed through the hallway. Doctors, nurses and other people walked around us. It felt like a dream; I was in a narrow tunnel where nobody could see me. The only thing real was the warmth and firmness of Daddy's hand.

I got iced tea, as that was "authorized"; it had no calories. Daddy got coffee and we sat down. I didn't want to look at him for fear of crying again. Daddy stirred cream and sugar into his coffee.

The cream swirled into the blackness, and my mind did the same. What was this monster that had overtaken me? Diabetes meant being controlled and maneuvered by many people, not the least of whom was my mother. Janis could do nothing without Mom knowing it, planning it, worrying and usually getting panicky over it. Mom had died a thousand deaths over my sister's well being. Somehow it worked for Mom and Janis. You'd think it might work for me. You would be wrong. That kind control was like a pillow over my face.

We sat a long time. Visiting hours were over, and the cafeteria was empty. Daddy finished seven cups of coffee, and I downed three glasses of iced tea. It was time to go back to the Hell Hole.

As we trudged back Daddy took my hand. It felt good, but I knew I had to figure out how to get along without it. I pulled my hand away. Dangling by my side, it went cold and numb.

"You okay?"

"Sure."

Then we were There.

He gave me a hug. "You gonna be okay?"

"Sure, Daddy." I sat on the bed, too heavy to stand.

He kissed me. "You get to go to school tomorrow. That'll be good."

"Yeah." Neither of us believed it.

"Remember I love you, sweetheart."

Tears burned in my eyes, but I wouldn't let them come out. Not this time. "I know."

He hugged me again and walked to the door, where he stopped and turned around. I knew he wanted to say something, do something. There was nothing to say or do.

I tried to smile.

So did he, then he was gone. While I was in the hospital he would stay with an old college friend who lived in Columbia. My bet was they would drink a lot of coffee, and talk late into the night over my new "situation". I wished I could be there drinking coffee with them.

It was up to me now. I stood up. The Vampire Squad would be coming for my blood first thing tomorrow morning. I had to be ready. I laid out my clothes. My red and brown plaid dress would be best, as I looked very grown up in it, and Mom said it made me look slender. People might be less apt to take advantage of a girl who looked slender and grown up. Black Sunday shoes, white socks...I was ready.

I put on my pink nightgown with the matching robe that Mom had gotten for me. Grown-ups wore matching gown and robe sets. I did all the things I would have done at home: brushed my teeth, washed my face, read my Bible. The routine was soothing.

Outside streetlights glimmered dimly through the rain-streaked windows, and the icy sleet still fell. *God, I need You more than I ever have in all my life. I need You all night, and especially when the needle people come in the morning.*

I was pretty sure He heard me, so I lay down. Tears threatened again, but I turned them to ice. There would be no more crying. Tomorrow I would be in control.

Lessons Learned:
1. Visiting hours are a form of hospital torture.
2. Strength and love flow through hugs.
3. Sometimes no amount of trying can stop tears.
4. Being grown up and slender is safer than little and fat.
5. God probably hears me, even if I say *damn*.

CHAPTER 4

Control held my only hope of survival. If I controlled what I ate, when and how long I exercised, took my insulin, did my urine tests, and wrote everything down in my record sheets, then I would be in control of my diabetes. That's what the doctors said. Keeping diabetes in control also meant I would have control over criticism from the doctors, my parents, and the world-in-general, which might make life bearable.

Appropriately enough, the Vampire Squad arrived in my room before dawn. I was not up and prepared as planned. With no other choice I proffered my arm, and the needle pierced my skin with a sharp slice. There was no further gouging or prodding; they must have gotten what they came for. She, the head Vampire, released the tourniquet and slid the needle from my arm. It was over.

Thank You, God, I thought. If only the idiot of yesterday could have been so skilled.

When the Vampires left, I got up. I was deadly calm. My first order of business was to go to the bathroom and catch my urine in the designated steel pitcher. I would now do this every day *for the rest of my life.* I showered and put on my grown up clothes. Methodically, I attended to every detail of hygiene and hair arrangement. I sat down to wait for the nurse who would take me to test my urine and go to the shot room.

She came.

I had transmographied (either I made up that word or read it somewhere) into a robot. As I walked down the hall with steel pitcher in hand, I realized the likeness; I had turned to steel.

The mixture in my test tube turned green, which meant my urine tested one percent. That was not good enough. It had to be "negative"…free from sugar, which was navy blue. I had to make blue show up. When it happened enough, it would be my ticket out of here.

We walked toward the shot room. The nurse chatted about something, and outwardly I said all the right things, smiled at the right times, and laughed appropriately. My freedom would come in playing the appropriate character for every role they threw at me. I would surpass their expectations. It might free me sooner.

We reached the shot room. I looked at the orders for my insulin dose, and drew it up in the syringe, mixing the long-acting and short-acting insulins together. I would have to inject myself today. Thinking about it had made my stomach churn all morning. The ocean was inside me, and the tide was going out.

I held the syringe and placed the needle on my leg. After many unsuccessful pricks, bruising, blood, and several lifetimes of anguish, I shoved the needle into my leg. The rest was easy.

I walked back to my room in a daze and sat down to wait for breakfast. My face and neck were cold and clammy. The tears I held captive had escaped as cold sweat.

Breakfast came, and along with it came Mrs. Margolis, the dietitian. That is what her nametag read. She was a big woman, tall and large-boned. She had gray hair wound into a tight bun, pinned perfectly in the center of the back of her head. Her face was wrinkled, but it looked soft. Her powder and lipstick gave her a "finished" look - not like a model, more like someone who always did the right thing, at the right place, at the right time.

"We've given you one meat exchange, one bread exchange, one fat exchange, one fruit exchange, and one milk exchange for breakfast. As you can see."

I definitely did not see. I looked at my tray. There was a boiled egg, a piece of toast with butter, an orange and a glass of milk. Okay, I did see. All those years of watching Mom prepare Janis' food had paid off. I knew what she was talking about.

"I see."

Mrs. Margolis looked surprised. "You do?" She straightened herself and looked even taller.

I wondered if she was German. I thought back to school, reading in history about German Nazis. It seemed to fit. "Yes. The egg is one meat exchange, the toast is the bread exchange, the butter is the fat exchange, the orange is the fruit exchange and the milk is the milk exchange." I looked up from the meal tray.

If she had looked surprised before, she now looked dumbfounded.

"My mom used to teach home economics, and she's made my sister's meals since before I was born. My sister has diabetes. What else do we need to go over?"

Mrs. Margolis stepped backward, and looked at me sideways. She seemed blown away. Good, that put me in control.

She walked to my bed and sat down, pulling out a small white booklet with black print. "You seem pretty up on this. You'll have it down in no time. After school today we'll have a lesson on all the different foods in the exchange lists, calorie levels, and meal planning. I'll see you then." She smiled, and her eyes twinkled.

Maybe she wasn't a Nazi after all.

When she left I ate breakfast without further interruptions, and a small song quietly played in my heart. I might make it through this; it all depended on being in control.

"Hello...?" The door opened a crack, and a dark-haired woman popped around the edge. "I'm Karen, and I'll be your nurse this morning." She was young, and had a nice smile.

Thank goodness she had a *real* name: not Dr. So-and-so or Mrs. Whatever, but *Karen.* "Hello. I'm Rachel Gifford." (Clever comeback...as if she didn't know that already.)

"Hi, Rachel. We'll be moving you to a ward across the hall today. I can do that for you while you're in school. Is that okay?"

I appreciated her asking my permission more than she could ever know. "I guess so, but I don't understand why you're moving me."

She looked around the room. "You're kind of alone in here. There are other girls in the ward, so you'll have company. You might like it better."

"Oh." Maybe I would, maybe I wouldn't. So much had been thrown at me; I was just getting used to my cell.

She smiled a really nice smile. Might I be able to trust her?

I made a quick decision. "Let's move stuff right now so I can help." I would have more control by helping than if they just up-and-moved everything while I was gone.

"Well, you need to go to school right now, so that won't work. I'll be careful with your things, though, and have you moved before lunch. We can talk then if you have any questions."

My trust dwindled. It's not like I had a lot to move, but what I had, was *all* I had in this place. What if she wrinkled my new dresses? What if she lost my socks? What if she plundered the birthday money Granny gave me before I left home?

She noticed my trepidation. "Tell you what...I'll let the teachers know you'll be a little late for school. Then we'll pile your stuff on the bed and move it into the ward. What d'ya think?"

"Good plan."

She winked and darted out the door toward the schoolroom.

I piled most of my things on the bed, leaving my dresses in the closet. I would carry them myself while Karen pushed the bed.

"Hi, Rachel. I'm back. Mrs. Bradshaw said it was fine for you to be a little late." She looked at my laden bed. "Oh, you're all ready!" Karen was the second person I'd surprised that morning, and it was barely eight a.m.

"Yep. Let's get going." I carefully took my dresses out of the closet. Karen positioned the bed for our trek across the hall. We nearly ran over a couple of doctors on the way. That was a bonus. Karen flashed me a grin, and we paraded on down the hall toward the ward.

The ward was a large room with places for eight beds, all of which were empty; probably the kids were at school? It was too open and non-private for my liking. The only privacy between beds was a curtain that could be drawn. The floor was slick, cold linoleum. The one impressive thing was the potential for friends and comrades-in-arms. I hung my dresses in the closet nearest my bed, and grabbed my notebook.

"See you at lunchtime, Karen!" Hurrying down the hall toward the schoolroom, I resumed worrying, this time about school. My grades always had been at the top of my class, but that was in my small-town school. What if I was behind all the pupils in the hospital and looked like an idiot? There went my control. I pushed the thought away, and quickened my pace toward the schoolroom.

Slowly I pushed the door open, and saw a woman at the blackboard. I decided she must be Mrs. Bradshaw. She was writing something that looked like a literature lesson. Mrs. Bradshaw was a medium-sized lady with brown-gray hair. She did not seem terribly scary, so I relaxed a few notches. I found a chair at a table with two other students.

Mrs. Bradshaw turned around. "You must be Rachel." She sounded fairly happy that I must be.

It helped.

"Let's take a moment to introduce ourselves. We've been waiting to do that until you arrived."

She was pleasant about the introduction thing, but quite frankly, I wished she would just continue with literature. Nevertheless, we all introduced ourselves and told what grade we were in. There were six other students in the room, and the age range was broad, from second to eighth grade. How in the world would we learn anything with such a mish-mash of grades?

Mrs. Bradshaw continued with literature. It was directed at my level, sixth grade – that was a relief. After literature was history, both subjects I liked. Then Mrs. Bradshaw dismissed the other kids for lunch, and asked me to stay a few minutes to go over my books from home. I was glad for personal attention, without the peering eyes of other kids.

"Where are you in each of your books, Rachel?" Mrs. Bradshaw peered at me over her reading glasses. She looked about Mom's age, and as she leafed through my books I noticed her soft hands. The kind of hands you would want to give you a snuggle or a pat on the cheek. I stopped her at the pages I last studied.

"This shouldn't be a problem at all. We can easily keep you up to date with your classmates."

"Thank you." I cleared my throat. "It'll be good not to be behind when I get back to school...whenever that finally happens."

She smiled. Her eyes were soft, and brown like mine. "We'll have you ahead of your class at home. It'll be easier for you to move ahead with personal attention. You'll have to wait for your friends to catch up once you're back home." She patted my arm with her soft hand. "We'll have fun, too. School here might be more fun."

She knew exactly what to say.

Back in the hallway, I spotted Karen. "Rachel, how was school?"

"Pretty good. Mrs. Bradshaw thinks I'll learn faster here than I did at my school at home."

"A lot of kids do. Mrs. Bradshaw's a good teacher. She's a nice lady, don't you think?"

"Yes, I do." And I certainly did.

"Let's go meet your new roommates." Karen took my hand and we walked to the ward.

There were four other girls. Theresa's bed was to my left. She had very long thick, dark, wavy hair. It was beautiful. She was drawing a picture of Cher.

"That's amazing! I can't draw at all, but your drawing looks just like the one in your magazine!"

Theresa beamed. "I really like to draw. It's a fun way to pass time."

I wondered how much time she'd been passing in the hospital.

Jenny and Patricia faced my bed from across the aisle, Patricia was closest to the door. I was farthest from the door, beside a wall of windows. Both Patricia and Jenny had diabetes, and were near my age. They had been diagnosed with diabetes for a while, but were having trouble with their blood sugar control. They were hospitalized for "re-regulation".

The thought sent icy fingers up my spine. It had not occurred to me that once I got out I might have to come back. I made a decision - I would not be back in this hospital again. Ever.

Susi's bed was directly across from me. She was just a child, maybe about six years old. She had blond hair and blue eyes, and her mom sat close by as Susi played with her dolls. She reminded me of the little kids Janis baby-sat. She did not look sick at all, but Karen said she was going to have surgery.

School went well in the afternoon. Lessons flew by, and even math was more fun than usual. After math we got to draw or read for a half hour. I read my Cherry Ames book. Cherry Ames and the Hardy boys were my favorite mystery stories, and since Cherry was a nurse, reading it in the hospital gave me a new perspective. Quite frankly, nearly everything about the hospital gave me a new perspective. I could fully understand why Cherry Ames was always coming across a dead body.

After school Jenny, who was a very take-charge kind of person, said she would introduce me to our evening nurse. "Her name is Madison, but everybody calls her Maddie. She is absolutely the best! ...graduated from nursing school last year; she's young and with-it. She'll even style your hair if you want. She let me use some of her make-up, too. She is absolutely *the* best!"

I could hardly wait to meet her. As soon as Maddie walked out of the nurse's station, I spotted her. She was tall and slender, but not skinny; more of an athletic build. Her hair was really short, dark brown, and thick, and she didn't wear a nurse's cap. Her hair glistened with a reddish hue when she walked under the fluorescent lights in the hallway. She wore a white uniform, white hose and white nursing shoes, but it didn't make her look dowdy or prissy. Instead, she looked like a model for a nursing ad. She definitely was with-it.

Jenny pulled me over to Maddie. "Hi, Maddie. This is Rachel. She just came yesterday."

Maddie looked down at me, but she didn't look down *on* me. She had freckles over her nose. I always wanted freckles, but Mom said girls with my coloring don't get them.

"Hi Maddie."

"Hi, Rachel." Her voice was energetic. She sounded like she could run a mile and not be tired.

"Rachel has diabetes, like me. But she's just been diagnosed. This is her first school day, so she doesn't know about running stairs or doing beauty parlor or snacks or any of the other good stuff."

Maddie smiled with the shiniest white teeth I'd seen in my life. "Wow. We need to show you."

I was more than ready.

Jenny motioned to me. "Come on! Let's go do urine tests so we'll be ready for dinner. Maddie, will you watch us and record our values?"

"Sure."

We got our urine pitchers and walked down the hall together. My pitcher still felt like steel, but I felt less metallic. Jenny had a one percent test, meaning her sugar was a little too high. Mine was negative. I was ecstatic!

"Maddie, since my urine is negative, does that mean I'll be going home soon?" I tried to keep the jubilation out of my voice, not wanting Jenny to feel bad.

"Are you wanting to go home soon?"

I cleared my throat. "Um.....yes. As soon as possible."

"Having a negative urine test is a good start. They usually have newly diagnosed diabetics stay in the hospital for a couple of weeks, so you can get all the education you need to take care of yourself when you go home."

My stomach tightened. "I just thought if my regulation went well, I might get out sooner."

"You know, Rachel, this place might not be so bad after you kind of get used to it." Maddie's eyes looked straight into my soul.

I hoped and prayed she was right.

Lessons Learned:
1. Being in control was my ticket home.
2. When you don't know what to do, play the role you're tossed.
3. Meal planning is a piece of cake, when you've watched your mom do it all your life.
4. So far, nurses and teachers in the hospital are kind, but the jury is still out.

CHAPTER 5

Dad came. I had eaten supper, and sat on my bed using the food exchange list to plan my menus. It was pretty easy. In fact it was kind of fun. I looked at my menu card to see how many exchanges of each food-type I was allowed then looked at the hospital menu sheets for each meal, and chose the food containing those exchanges. The only tricky part was when casseroles were on the menu, because they had several food-types in them. I had to consult my manual from Mrs. Margolis on those.

"How's it going, punkin?"

Dad called me punkin' when he was happy. I had not heard it for a while. Maybe we were both coming around.

"Whaddya doin'?" He looked at my pile of papers.

"Marking menu sheets for the next several days. Mrs. Margolis showed me how."

"Does anybody help you on this?"

"Nope. Mrs. Margolis checks them after I finish, but so far I've only messed up a couple a things."

Dad sat on the chair by my bed, and looked pleased. "Ya' know, that's really good."

"Thanks. Hey! You know what else? My urine test was *negative*!" I felt warm inside. Maybe I *could* do all this stuff: shots, food exchanges, turning my pee blue. If Dad thought I could, it was a start.

"Mail call!" Maddie strolled in with a bunch of envelopes in her hand.

Jenny jumped off her bed and held out her hand.

"Two for you, Jenny! One for Patricia, and Theresa you win the Mail Prize today with four, count them - one...two...three...four letters!" She grinned and handed them out.

Darn. Sure, this was only Day Two for me, but it would have been nice to get something.

"Well, and look at this. One for Rachel! Somebody sure loves you, they mailed you a letter the day you got here."

"Thanks!" I snatched the letter. "It's from Granny!" I looked at Dad.

His smile said he was not at all surprised.

I ripped open the envelope. She not only sent a card, but a two page letter, and three one-dollar bills. "Dad, look at this!" I waved my bounty.

"You hit the jackpot, punkin!"

I sat down and looked at the card from front to middle to back four times. It was bright pink, and on the front it said, "I can't imagine someone as wonderful as you being sick." On the inside it said, "I guess that means you'll be better soon!" I sniffed it. It smelled like Granny. She wore Evening in Paris perfume, because that's what all of her six grandchildren bought her for Christmas. With every package she opened, she would exclaim, "It's my favorite perfume!" We were glad, because on a kid's allowance, it was the only one we could afford, and still have money to spread around for the rest of the family. I envisioned Granny with the little dark blue bottle, putting a dab behind each ear. A sniffle threatened. I sat up very straight and threw my head back – the tears stopped.

Dad looked over. "You okay?"

"Sure, fine. Neat card from Granny. Wanna see it?"

He reached for the card.

I started reading the letter. Granny had kind of scrawly handwriting. Sometimes it was a little hard to read, but it looked beautiful. She said she and Grandpa were very sad about my diabetes, but they knew I would be absolutely okay very soon, and I would be able to take care of myself.

Tears began to build.

She went on to say my cousin, Tommy, had stopped by to visit her and get the cookies, cake and cinnamon rolls she made for him to take back to college. I smiled. Granny made the best oatmeal scotchies in the world. The only thing better was her homemade chocolate cake with chocolate fudge icing. She usually made too much icing for the cake, and put the extra on top in big dollops. (That was her word.) I picked off the dollops first like hunks of chocolate fudge, and then went for the cake. Thinking about it made my mouth water.

Then it hit me - my dollop days were over. Dollops were not on the Exchange List. The list included angel food cake. Who cares about angel food cake? My tear reservoir broke through the dam. If I couldn't have Granny's chocolate cake there was no point in having more birthdays. Tears skied down my nose and splatted onto Granny's letter.

"Rachel...? Are you okay?" Daddy looked at me.

"No. I will never be okay again."

"What?"

I handed him the letter.

He read for a little while, then looked up at me. "Granny says Tommy's coming to visit you Thursday evening. Only two days off."

"What!" I forgot the dollops. Tommy was my favorite cousin in the whole world. He was eight years older than me, and the coolest guy in existence....next to Dad, of course. He had wavy black hair and snappy dark eyes that were full of mischief. Tommy was tall and lean, and always looked like he had the world in the palm of his hand. Just imagining his grin made me chuckle. He loved to hunt and fish, and always caught really big fish. One day he and one of his buddies were trying to shoot a bird off the telephone wire, and shot right through the wire! That was a hard one to explain to the phone company.

Being ornery suited him well, and he got into a bit of trouble from time to time, which just made him more fun. I could not believe he was going to drive all the way from Kirksville, Missouri, two hours away, just to come see me. Even on Thursday, a school night. Wow.

"We have to call and find out what time he's coming. I want to be sure I'm done with all my testing, menu planning, studies and everything." I jumped off the bed and scanned my clothes closet. The brown slacks and blue blouse with the brown window-pane pattern and Peter Pan collar would be best. It looked grown-up and "together"; not too dressy, not too casual.

My heart pounded. Oh, my gosh. This *almost* made it worth being here. Of course I could see Tommy nearly any day of the week at home, but this was different. Here I had him all to myself. I would get Maddie to do the beauty shop and make-up thing Jenny told me about. I ran to find her.

"Maddie!" I sprinted to the doorway of the nurse's station. "My cousin, Tommy, is coming to visit Thursday evening! Can you do my hair? Jenny says you're fantastic. Can you help me with some make-up? This is really important, Maddie. This is beyond important. It's *GRANDIOSE!*" I looked at her expecting she would understand everything, and have an answer that would match my enthusiasm.

"Uh...yeah...tell me a little more about this Grandiose Event."

"Sure!" I spilled the story in just over one breath.

"Find out what time he's coming on Thursday, and we'll be sure you're gorgeous!"

"Thanks! Jenny is right. You are *the* best."

Maddie grinned.

I grinned back, and floated to my room.

"Dad, we have to call Mom!"

"Okay, but we can't talk long, because...."

"I know, because it's expensive."

"Right."

I grabbed his hand and pulled him toward the hall phone. He called, and I could hear Mom's voice on the line. They talked about this and that, but did not get to the important question.

"Ask her what time Tommy is coming, Dad. Find out what time on Thursday."

He looked at me absent-mindedly and shook his head up and down.

I waited.

They talked.

"Dad, this call is getting expensive. Ask her what time Tommy is coming." That got his attention.

"Seven-thirty? Okay. Rachel is really looking forward to it. Bye, hon. I love you. Kiss Holly and Janis for me. Bye." He hung up.

"Seven-thirty?"

"Seven-thirty."

"Soooooo cool!"

Would Thursday ever come?

Wednesday morning dawned, and I realized the Vampire Squad had not come for me. It was strange, but I certainly was not going to mention it to anyone. My pee was blue again. My final frontier were the shots.

Giving shots was really hard. Drawing up the insulin and mixing it was easy. Stabbing that needle into my body was nearly more than I could do. They gave me choices: arm, thigh, abdomen or hip, making it sound as if I was choosing between chocolate cake, ice cream, cookies or banana cream pie. Had they completely lost touch with reality? I would have preferred to use *their* arm, thigh, abdomen or hip, but it did not work that way.

In the shot room I finally stabbed the needle into my hip, injected the insulin, and went back to the ward. Jenny had done her shot at the same time, so we walked together.

"Jenny, does this ever get easier?"

"It gets less scary after awhile, but it hurts, and sometimes it bleeds a lot and gets on your clothes. It's hard when other people are around, because they think you're doing drugs, and give you weird looks."

"I never thought about that. Are you scared a lot?"

"Yeah." We walked a few steps in silence. "One time," Jenny said, "my mom told me about this guy who was driving and had an insulin reaction. He had a wreck, and the police thought he was drunk. Instead of getting him medical help, they put him in jail, and when they went to get him the next morning, he was dead."

I stopped walking. The gravity of what she said stuck my feet to the floor. "They didn't help him? They let him die?"

"They didn't know he had diabetes." She held up her arm. "That's why I always wear this." A large, very ugly silver ID bracelet hung on her wrist. On the top of it was a big red symbol and the word *DIABETIC*.

"You wear that all the time?"

"Yep."

"Even when you go to bed?"

"Yeah. My doctor said you never know when an emergency could happen, and people need to know you have diabetes."

I couldn't take it in. It reminded me of when Dad and Grandpa branded cattle, so no one could mistake them for belonging to someone else. For the rest of my life, I would be branded *DIABETIC* with a big ugly bracelet.

"What about the shots? It takes me ten or fifteen minutes to get up enough courage to stab myself with that needle. Does that ever get better?" I wanted her to say it got really easy after awhile, but I had my doubts.

"Well, sometimes I just don't give my shots."

"What!?" I gaped at her. "Whadda you mean? Is that okay to do?"

"No, not really. That's why I'm back in the hospital. My sugar goes really high. I tell my mom I took my shots and I don't know why my sugar is high. She calls the doctor, and I end up here again."

I was in shock. The doctors had told me shots would keep me alive now that I had diabetes. They said if I did not take shots, test my urine and follow my exchange diet I would go blind, have to have my legs cut off because of gangrene (whatever that was), and have to go on dialysis. They jabbed it in my face like a threat. I had heard it at least twice a day since getting here.

"You have *got* to be kidding! You'll die. Don't you know that?"

Jenny's lips formed a gentle smile. "You know, the doctors tell you that to scare you. The first year I had diabetes I ran scared every minute of every day. I thought if I didn't do everything perfect like they said, I'd die. Not only that, one doc would tell me one thing, and next time I'd go back to the clinic a different doc would tell me something different. They both said if I didn't do exactly what they said, I'd ruin my health. They sounded real stupid after a while. This is my life. I've got to live it my way, and they don't want to help me. They just want to sound off." She leaned toward my face. "You know, I'd just like to see one of them do all the crap they tell us to do, for just one week. They'd fall on their butts!" She giggled. "And they threaten us, thinking it will make us 'be good' for the *rest of our lives!*" She bent over and howled with laughter.

Icy fingers ran down my spine. But Jenny's laughter was contagious, pretty soon we were leaning on each other for strength. Then we leaned against the wall and slid down, sitting cross-legged on the cold tile floor as we gasped for breath. It was a long time before we got up.

Lessons Learned:

1. Planning menus isn't hard, but it's more of a hassle than just eating.
2. Stabbing myself with a needle is nearly impossible. The rest of shot-giving is easy.
3. Laughing pushes fear out the backdoor of my heart.

CHAPTER 6

"Rachel, I understand you recently had a birthday." Mrs. Bradshaw pulled me aside as we took a break after literature.

"Yes, I did." I didn't care to go into it. As birthdays go, it had been crummy.

"Well, we'd like to help you celebrate it."

This was not good news. There would be no chocolate cake and Granny wouldn't be there.

"What did you have in mind? I can't have cake or ice cream, you know."

"Yes, I know. But Mrs. Margolis can help us come up with something really tasty."

She was trying to be nice, but this would not work. "Mrs. Bradshaw, it might be better to just wait until next year."

She gave me an earnest look. "Rachel, birthdays are special, and I'd like for you to feel special. We'll have something nice this afternoon during our break."

So it was final. One would think I would be able to have the final say in celebrating my birthday. One would be wrong. Having a birthday with angel food cake was a joke. I'd just as soon eat styrofoam. And how could I possibly celebrate in this sterile prison, with people I didn't even know?

Yet, she had a point, celebrating was important. Maybe it would make me feel better. I doubted it.

As I ate my morning snack of fruit and milk, I told Patricia what Mrs. Bradshaw had said. She was ecstatic.

"Rachel, that is *so* cool! Parties are good, ya know. Besides, maybe we'll do it during geography. That is *such* a boring class!"

She obviously didn't get it. Yet, maybe in some way it would make up for what I was going through. A tiny hope glimmered in my brain.

"Hey, Rachel, Lonnie wants to see you," Theresa said. She was sketching pictures from her Seventeen magazine during the break.

"What does she want?" I felt anxious. Heaven only knew what was up now.

"Dunno. Didn't seem like a really big deal. I think she said something about an x-ray."

"X-ray?" At least it didn't involve a needle.

"Yeah. She's at the nurse's station. Go check it out."

"Okay." I headed toward the nurse's station. Lonnie was standing outside the station, writing on a chart.

"Hi Lonnie. You need me?"

"Hi, Rachel. Yes, we need to do a chest x-ray on you this afternoon. It's a standard procedure for each new admit. Just a precaution."

"For what?"

"Tuberculosis. If you had it we'd catch it early, and keep other people from being exposed."

"I don't have tuberculosis. I have diabetes." This place got stupider by the minute.

She laughed. "I know. It's just routine. No needles. They just take a picture of your chest. We can do it this afternoon."

I remembered the birthday party. "Mrs. Bradshaw and my class are having a birthday party for me this afternoon at our two o'clock break. Can I do the x-ray tomorrow?"

Lonnie looked up from charting. "Oh, it won't take long, Rachel. You'll be back in plenty of time. That's really nice to have a party!"

Famous last words. Nothing in this place happened fast, and I was sure the x-ray people wouldn't give a flip about my birthday party. Suddenly the party held more importance. "Are you *sure* I'll be able to do the party? I don't think I'll be back in time."

"Sure you will. When we go to x-ray, we'll let them know you need to be back in time for your party. We'll go right after lunch."

Maybe she was right. Maybe not. Does anybody in this place ever listen?

After lunch we headed to x-ray. I memorized the way, so I could get back to the floor without help if I needed to make a quick exit.

"This is Rachel Gifford, here for a chest x-ray." Lonnie signed me in at the front desk. "Rachel, you can sit right over here. They'll call your name in a few minutes."

"Did you tell them I have to be back upstairs no later than two o'clock?"

"Oh, I forgot! I'll let them know." She walked back to the check-in desk, and talked with the receptionist. The receptionist nodded, and Lonnie walked to the elevator.

I nodded at the receptionist.

She smiled, and disappeared behind the counter.

I sat. After a while I looked at my watch: one-twenty. My stomach got jumpy. I didn't know how long the x-ray took, but time was getting short. I walked to the check-in counter. "Excuse me?"

Nothing.

I mustered my gumption and proclaimed to the faceless counter, "EXCUSE ME!"

A face appeared above the counter. It was the receptionist. "Yes?"

"Upstairs in my schoolroom they will have a birthday party, for me, at two o'clock sharp. I want to be there for my party. Can you help me?" My palms were sweating.

"Oh, I'm sure it will be all right, dear. They're very busy doing x-rays on other people right now. They'll get to you."

"You don't understand. I have a deadline." A wad of anger grew in my stomach.

She gave me an irritated glance. "If you'd like, you can change into a gown in the dressing room so you don't waste time when they're ready for you."

Great, another strip-tease gown, but it might speed things along. "Okay. Where are the dressing rooms?"

She led me to a back area, handed me a gown and showed me to a small room.

"Do I come back out to the waiting room after I change?" I hoped not.

"No. Just wait here in the room."

That was not much better. The changing room was the size of a phone booth and had no windows. It was a cage where you would keep small helpless creatures before butchering and eating them.

I changed into the gown, and carefully folded my own clothes, putting them neatly in a pile. I sat down to wait. Fifteen more minutes escaped: one thirty-five. I opened the door a crack and peered into the hallway. No one in sight. I sat back down and waited another five minutes. I was dangerously close to missing the party.

I opened the door; still no one in the hallway. I gathered my gown in the back to limit exposure, and walked to the check-in counter.

"Excuse me, Ma'am."

The receptionist's head rose above the counter not unlike a magical resurgence of the Loch Ness monster.

"I have only twenty minutes to get an x-ray, get dressed and back to my classroom for my birthday party. Pleeeeeeease, can you help me?"

She gave me the look my mom uses on my brother when he waits under his bed in the dark, and jumps out shooting her with his cap gun. "Child! We have sick people here who need care. They are more important than a party. I'll check with the doctors, and in the meantime, Go. Sit. Down."

I sat down. At least my body sat down. My mind raced after her yelling, "I *am* important, and so is my birthday!" I wanted to tell her she was rude, mean and generally a nasty, insensitive lady. But I didn't. I sat quietly. Anger swelled past my stomach and into my chest on its way to my throat.

The receptionist returned and sat down hard in her chair. It squeaked loudly in protest. It was now one forty-five. This was the second birthday jerked out from under me in less than a week. It must be some kind of record. I hated this woman. I hated this place that gave no validity to humanity. I hated these people who daily reduced my worth to less than road kill. I hated their ignoble tolerance of me. I hated being in their control, and not in my own. I hated this situation, and this new life that had taken over everything I ever used to know. I stood up and marched stiffly to the dressing room. I would put on my own clothes and go to my party, leaving this place and their damn x-ray. As I changed I heard a knock on the door.

"Miss Giffer?" A female voice spoke through the door.

"What."

"Miss Giffer we are ready to do your x-ray."

"It's too late, I don't have time."

There was a pause. "Miss Giffer, we *have to do your x-ray!*" The voice beseeched and demanded at the same time.

I paused. My watch said 1:55 p.m.. Anger had reached my head, and was drilling a ditch in the left side.

"I only have five minutes before my party."

"Oh, no problem, Miss Giffer. We can have you back in five minutes!"

She was lying. I even knew *she* knew she was lying. I was powerless against this Medical Machine. I wanted to climb to the top of the Medical Center with a loudspeaker and scream to the world, *"Every White Coat inside this building is a dirty, rotten, big-fat-liar!"*

I put the gown back on and walked into the hall. We went to the x-ray room. As I waited for the x-ray to be taken, and then developed, I knew everyone upstairs in my classroom was enjoying my birthday party. The Medical Machine had triumphed, but the patient had died.

Finally I was done. I changed clothes and returned to the floor. It was two forty-five; only fifteen minutes left in the school day. I walked slowly to the schoolroom, to see if anything was left of the party I didn't have.

Mrs. Bradshaw sat at her desk doing paperwork. She looked up as I opened the door. "Rachel! I'm so glad you're here. I'm sorry you didn't get to have your party today. Your angel food cake and scoop of ice cream are here. Would you like them?"

I looked at the melted glob of ice cream soaking into the styrofoam cake, in a wilting paper bowl. "No, thank you, Mrs. Bradshaw. Was it a good party?"

She bit her lip. "Rachel, I'm sorry about the x-ray schedule. That kind of thing happens a lot around here. We'll have another party for you."

"No, Mrs. Bradshaw, we will not. My birthday is over for this year." There would be no more discussion of birthdays or parties. I closed the door and walked to the ward.

"Hey, Rachel, sorry about the party." It was Patricia.

"Yeah." I walked past her and sat on my bed.

It was a gray bleak day outside, and the sun already was low in the sky. February definitely had short days. Abraham Lincoln probably had some bad birthdays on his February twelfths, too. Especially with his mom dying, the Civil War, and losing two of his children, and all.

I looked across the room toward Susi's bed. It was freshly made. Susi had gone to her mysterious surgery sometime after lunch, looking as cute and healthy as she had when I first saw her. Her mother had not looked so good, though. She looked tense. The way Mom looked on mornings after Janis had insulin reactions. Life outside these hospital walls seemed an eternity away, yet this was only Day Three.

Maddie came bustling in. She rushed to Susi's bed and pulled back the covers. "Susi's here!" She zoomed back to the hallway.

A gurney wobbled into the ward pushed by numerous white clad people, and accompanied by several more pushing IV poles and paraphernalia of all sorts. There was much beeping and clanking. I couldn't see Susi. She was buried beneath piles of blankets....white, of course. What an odd, nervous, mechanical procession.

They wheeled to Susi's bed, where a white clad guy picked up her limp little body and slid it from gurney to bed. They put a bunch of blue pads underneath her for "drainage." I wasn't sure what was draining, but it did not sound pleasant. There were tubes attached to her arms that I assumed were IV stuff, she had cords coming out the top of her hospital gown, and a big tube attached to a bag full of bright red fluid (blood?) that hung from her bed. All this on such a tiny girl.

Susi's face matched the mound of blankets covering her. She'd become a ghost of her former self. A blue cap covered her golden curls. I felt sick. Susi was not recognizable as the little girl who left our room just a few hours before. Was she dying?

Susi's mother did not look much better, except she didn't have tubes and wires. She took the blue cap off Susi's head and wiped her forehead with a washcloth. Susi started throwing up. Maddie grabbed a little half-circle pan and held it under Susi's mouth. Green stuff came out. I had never seen anything like this in my entire life; all twelve years of it. They drew the curtains around Susi's bed, but I could still hear her retching and moaning.

The gurney and most of the White Coats cleared out, leaving Maddie and Susi's mother to keep vigil over what was left of Susi. They pulled the curtains back and the sight of Susi made tears prickle behind my eyes. I wanted to help, but I had no idea how. This was indeed, a treacherous place.

Dinner came, but I was not hungry.

Dad walked in. "Hi punkin'. What's going on?"

I had hoped he could explain it to me. "Susi had surgery today, but something must have gone really wrong. I think she's dying." I whispered to him, because it was too morose to say out loud.

He looked surprised. "Why do you say that?"

"Well, *look* at her!"

He looked toward her bed, and nodded. "Not so good, but I don't think she's dying."

How could he possibly come to that conclusion?

"Mail call!" Several hours had passed, and Maddie had left Susi and her mother for other tasks. I got seven letters! Granny sent two and some friends from church and school sent the others. Molly, who used to be my best friend until this school year when she pretty much dumped me, sent one, and said everybody in class would be writing. Mrs. Barker, my teacher, was going to mail all of them on Saturday. Wow! I'd have tons of mail next week. I secretly hoped I might not be here to get it, but in my heart I knew it was a ruse. For thinkers, sometimes the brain says one thing and the heart says something different. At those times, usually the brain is lying.

Night came, and Dad left. I was getting used to the schedule. I no longer felt like I would die when he left. Susi was quiet now, and her mother looked a little better. The lights went down and we all slept.

"Mama! Mama!" It was Susi. The ward was dark, with only the hall light casting a dim glow. What time was it? I slid out of bed, put on my pink robe and slippers, and tip-toed across the room.

"Susi? It's me, Rachel. Are you okay?" I took her soft, tiny hand, holding only her fingers, so I wouldn't disturb the IV tubes.

"Maaaama.....Maaaamaaaaaa...."

I wanted to cry, too. God felt closer when I was alone, especially at night. *God, please help Susi.* I pulled Susi's call button, and stroked her forehead as I'd seen her mother do earlier. She became less restless. I curled my fingers around hers and sat down in the chair by her bed. Surely with praying and the call button, help would come before she died.

"Hello...?"

Someone gently shook my shoulder. I had fallen asleep in the chair. It was still dark, and Susi was making quiet snoring noises. A nurse I had never met before stood over me.

"What are you doing here?"

I rubbed my eyes. "Keeping Susi company. She was dy...er...crying."

"That's kind of you. I'll give her some medication and you can go back to bed."

I let go of Susi's fingers and shuffled toward my bed. Crawling in, I lay down and pulled up the covers. *Please God help Susi get better.*

Helping Susi had made me feel better...it reminded me I mattered.

Lessons Learned:

1. The Medical Machine has no soul. It doesn't care about people; it doesn't have a heart. It is the Living Dead.
2. Surgery is supposed to help you, but it may kill you.
3. Helping someone else helps me.
4. God often hovers in the dark. I'd prefer He just show up in the daylight.

CHAPTER 7

Thursday *finally* arrived. My day was planned to the last jot and tittle, to make sure I was ready for Tommy's visit. The anticipation was chocolate dollops for the brain. On occasion the unwelcome thought of his departure after the visit, came to mind. I glared it into submission with mental laser vision.

My agenda included school as usual, followed immediately by Maddie doing my hair and make-up. I had never worn make up before, so the importance of this visit continued to mount. Homework was on the docket while I ate dinner; I was an early pioneer to multi-tasking.

At seven p.m. I would change into my brown slacks, and the light blue shirt with brown window-pane print and Peter Pan collar. Then I would read mail until Tommy came, in hopes it would keep my mind busy enough to prevent going berserk while I waited.

"You ready for school?" Patricia had her books and was heading toward the door.

"Yeah, just a minute." I grabbed my books, and we started down the hall.

"Did you know Theresa is having surgery tomorrow?"

I stopped mid-stride. Visions of Theresa, lying in her bed looking as dead as Susi, flashed across my brain. "Who told you that?"

"Theresa."

"Is she scared?"

"Didn't seem like it. She's had four back surgeries, and I think she's got it down to a routine."

Theresa had told me she had something called a "scoliosis". It meant her back grew crooked, and they had to do surgeries to straighten her spine. She said they put a rod in her back, and every time she grew, they had to lengthen the rod. It sounded like a gruesome medieval torture, but Theresa had been calm as a clam when she told me.

"Do you think she'll look dead as Susi when she comes back?"

Patricia was quiet for several steps. "Don't know. She says she won't come back to our ward. They'll take her to ICU for a while. She may be a lot worse than Susi."

I tried to imagine a live human being looking worse than Susi. No picture came.

"Theresa says after the surgery she'll be in a "Stryker frame" or something like that. She said it's like a hammock, and every hour they put another hammock-thing on top of her, and turn her over. She'll be like a pancake getting flipped every hour until she's done."

"How long before she's done?"

"She said last time she was in the hospital a month."

"A *month*?!! Are you nuts? A person could *die* spending a whole month here."

"Yeah, well that's not even the worst of it. She says she has to be in a body cast for nine months to a year after she gets out."

"What?! How do you go to the bathroom? What about showers? How do you sit down? What about clothes?"

"Don't know you'll have to ask her. It's weird how much she knows."

My head spun. How could someone have something so wrong with them they had to continually go to the hospital and endure tortures? When did she go to school? How could she exist, knowing that in a few months she would have to start the whole process over?

Suddenly diabetes did not seem so bad. But who knew if what happened to Theresa might happen to me? These illnesses parading through our ward were no respecter of persons. There was adorable little Susi: one day looking just fine, the next day having surgery for some unknown reason, draining her very life's blood into a bag hanging on her bed and looking dead. Now Theresa had a life filled with ongoing horror. There were all the kids in our schoolroom in wheelchairs for various reasons, and the kids who had cancer and looked like they had been burned alive. Patricia, Jenny and I had a disease that could strike us down in unconsciousness or seizures at any moment, and ultimately might make us have our legs chopped off or go blind. And we didn't even look sick! Was the disease or the treatment worse? The violence flattened me.

Suddenly my stomach churned. "Patricia, I have to go to the bathroom. Tell Mrs. Bradshaw I'm coming."

"You okay? Whatever you do, don't puke. They'll have to start an IV."

"Right." I clamped my hand over my mouth and sprinted toward the hall bathroom. Patricia was right. I had been able to escape the morning Vampire Squad for two days in a row, and did not want an IV. Thoughts raced so fast I couldn't get to the end of one, before another swooped in like a hawk after a baby bunny.

I slammed the bathroom door and put my face against the cool metal. I had to rally.

I slid to the tile floor. *I will be okay. I will not throw up. I won't get an IV. My back isn't crooked, and I don't have to be sliced open every year. All I have to do is everything they tell me to, and I'll get out of here. With God as my witness, I will never ever, as long as I live, come back. Never.*

The cement mixer in my stomach ground to a halt. I sat quietly several minutes. I was steel again.

Standing up I looked in the mirror. My eyes and nose were red, and my face streaky. I wet paper towels and rubbed my cheeks. I pushed up the corners of my mouth and made them stay there. It was a mask, but nobody on the outside would be the wiser. If they didn't know, they wouldn't ask. If they didn't ask, I wouldn't tell. I'd get out of this House of Horrors, and be normal again.

It was a good story, but I knew the ending was a lie - nothing would ever be normal again. Slowly, quietly I walked toward the classroom. I opened the door, tip-toed in, and sat down. No one noticed I was a robot.

"Maddie, Maddie! Can you do my hair now?" School was out, and according to schedule, it was time for my coiffure.

Maddie walked out of the nurse's station as I rounded the corner. "Hey! How's it goin'?

"I'm ready to get beautiful."

"Let's get started." We headed toward the ward.

Maddie zipped into action, wrapping a towel around my shoulders just like Mom's beautician at home. She washed and rolled my hair, and sat me under a portable dryer borrowed from the hospital storeroom. While my hair dried, Patricia, Jenny and I looked at magazines and giggled. We had our own private beauty shop.

After much giggling and magazine looking, Maddie took off the dryer and unrolled a curler.

"You're done baking. Now for the styling magic of Maddie the Magnificent, most sought after beautician-nurse of all time!"

She combed, back-combed, styled and sprayed. I thought I might need a gas mask. Finally, she handed me a mirror.

"I can't believe it! My hair's never looked this good."

Maddie became French. "And now, Madam, for ze make-up." After several minutes, numerous dabs, blots and swishes, she handed back the mirror.

The girl looking back at me had a family resemblance, but that's where the similarity ended. She, in the mirror, was gorgeous. I, in the chair, was not. I looked down at my dress. Strangely enough, we both wore the same clothes.

"Maddie, why didn't you become a beautician instead of a nurse?"

"I wanted to do both. If I'd been a beautician, that's all I'd have gotten to do. This way, I get to be a nurse and beautician. Making people beautiful makes them feel better."

She had it figured out. I wished I had it figured out, but for now, looking gorgeous was good enough.

"Okay, now I have to get my homework done and eat."

"What a planner!" Maddie laughed.

I hoisted myself on the bed, and sat cross-legged, piling school books around me. Within minutes I was deep into social studies, reading the antics of various explorers, obsessed with finding new territories to claim for their homeland. I wondered how the world might be different if these guys had gotten real jobs and stayed home with their families. Would there have been fewer wars? Less killing? Would Indians and buffalo still roam free on the plains? Would our world today be a table top instead of a globe? These thoughts were neither queried nor answered in the scope of my books, making me doubt seriously if the author was much of a thinker.

Somewhere between the conquest of the Incas and the geographical description of South America, the thought of visiting with Tommy popped out of nowhere. Giggles overtook me. The reality submerged an abyss of unpleasantness. I shook myself and refocused on the topography of Peru.

After wading through the riches of Peru for some time, I was jolted out of cerebral travels by the clattering of the dinner cart. I retrieved my tray and checked to be sure it held all the correct exchanges, according to Mrs. Margolis' instructions. She said that after all, anybody can make mistakes, so I should double-check. Apparently I was not anybody - the buck stops here.

Dad strode in. "Hey, punkin', how's it going!" He let out what Mom calls a wolf whistle. "Look at you!"

"Hi, Dad. Maddie the Magnificent did it. Less than two hours before Tommy comes!"

"That's right," he said, glancing at his watch. "How's your homework?"

"Only three pages left to read, eat dinner, change clothes, read my mail, and voila! I'm ready." I hoped he realized my need to stay on schedule.

"Sounds like a plan." Dad liked being on schedule. Mom was never on schedule, and it always was a point of contention between them. It spread tension and yelling through every family member.

"Yep. I better read now." I blindly forked food into my mouth, while my brain returned to the flora and fauna of Peru. Why explorers would raid, pillage and imprison such an astounding land and people was beyond me. What were the Spanish thinking? But then, I saw it only in hindsight, and Granny says hindsight is always twenty-twenty. Anyway, none of this related to my life, on this day, when Tommy was coming to visit. Yet, the task was assigned, so it must be done. On schedule.

"I'll go get some coffee while you're doing your stuff. Want me here for your visit or do you want Tommy all to yourself?"

"You might want to go for a long coffee, Dad."

"You got it, punkin'." He kissed me and strode out the door.

How was it Dad always looked like he owned the world? Did he really feel that way? I wished I felt that way...even part of the time

At seven p.m. sharp my body sent out an alert. I had just finished the last assigned paragraph. I jumped off the bed and headed for the little locker I used as a closet, snatching out my brown pants, and blue blouse. Jerking the curtain around my bed, I changed clothes. I had to be careful not to mess up my hair or smudge the make-up. I caught my reflection in the mirror on my bedside table. I had never fantasized the word gorgeous as related to myself before, but quite frankly...I qualified. I was Cinderella.

I opened the curtain around my bed, and sat lady-like in the bedside chair - legs crossed at the ankle, feet tucked under the chair. Mom said that was how grown up ladies sat. I went through mail quietly and discreetly, reading each card, carefully refolding and replacing every letter back into the envelope, laying each envelope on my bed in a neat stack. It worked... my mind was staying with the mail.

"Rachel?" Maddie's voice broke my concentration.

"What!"

"Good grief, no need to yell. You have visitors." Her brown eyes danced teasingly.

I jumped from my grown up sitting position, caught my foot on the chair, and nearly fell on my face. "Cool! Let's go!"

"It's not Tommy. Sorry."

"What!" My heart sank to the floor.

"No. There are three young men down in the lobby to see you."

"Three? *Men?*"

"Yes, it seems cousin Tommy, of the Grandiose Event, has brought buddies with him. They're all awaiting your entrance in the lobby. Shall I escort you down?"

"Let's go!" I sprang for the door, and Maddie hustled along behind me. We rounded the nurse's station and closed in on the elevator at an undignified gallop. I pushed the button.

"...a little...excited?" Maddie leaned against the wall to catch her breath.

The elevator arrived and I pushed the lobby button before Maddie could get in. The door hit her shoulder and bounced back open.

"You're slowing things down!"

Maddie rolled her eyes and rubbed her shoulder.

I pushed the "Door Close" and "Nonstop" buttons. Cinderella was headed for the ball. The elevator squealed to a stop, and the doors parted. The lobby spread before me, and lo and behold....there was Tommy! He sat smack-dab in the middle under a big palm plant, with two other guys about his age. He jumped up as I ran toward him.

"Rachel!" He grabbed me in a bear hug, squashing my ribs. "My gosh, you look great."

My face got hot. "Yeah, Maddie did this."

Maddie stepped out from under the palm plant. "Hi, Tommy. Good to meet you. Rachel has been looking forward to your visit." She stuck out her hand.

Tommy shook it hard...too hard for gentlemanly manners.

Maddie didn't seem to mind.

Finally, he let go and turned to the guys on the couch. "This is Andy," he pointed to the guy on his left, "and Bill," he turned to the right. "It's a long drive, so my buddies came to help me."

I remembered Tommy's collection of speeding tickets that had been the chagrin of both his parents. Other drivers were a good idea. We all sat down except Maddie, who excused herself and headed toward the elevators.

Tommy leaned toward me. "So what's going on? How are they treating you here?"

"Wow, you can't even believe it." Tears swam to my eyes. Would he think I was a wimp and exaggerating how scary everything was? I told him anyway, about the Vampire Squad, school, all the sick kids, Susi and Theresa, surgery, and how people came back looking dead. I talked until my throat got hoarse.

"I don't know what to say." Tommy's eyes held tears.

"I know, neither do I." I looked away. "So...how's college?"

"Oh, it's good. I've got several eight o'clock classes. In fact I have one tomorrow morning that I might not make." He grinned. Tommy was known for missing a few classes. He talked more about college, and suddenly visiting hours were over. This really was like Cinderella.

He and his buddies stood up. For the first time, I noticed how much bigger he was than me. He was taller than Dad.

The tears returned to Capistrano. Tommy pulled out his handkerchief and handed it to me.

"Thanks." I wiped my eyes and handed it back with black mascara stains.

He dabbed his eyes. "I love you, Rachel."

"I love you, too."

We hugged, and three *men* walked into the night. All my joy went with them. The clock had struck midnight, the ball gown became rags, the coach was a pumpkin, and the fine white horses were street rats again.

After staring out the door at nothing for a small eternity, I turned toward the elevator. Between the elevator and me there was a snack bar I hadn't noticed before. Granny's three dollars were in my pocket, so I shuffled toward the counter. Maybe buying something would make me feel better.

I scanned the contents, looking for anything that said sugar-free. There it was - sugar-free gum. I bought cinnamon and peppermint, stuck the change in the pocket of my grown up brown slacks, and headed to my cell on the eighth floor. The elevator deposited me. The doors clanged shut. I walked slowly down the empty corridor, my steps echoing off the hard, cold walls.

I needed to be with a human. Visiting hours were over, so I knew Dad had gone. Maybe Maddie hadn't left for the night yet. I headed toward the nurse's station munching the cinnamon gum, hoping the peppery flavor could warm me. Maddie was gone, but Dr. Henry, one of the residents, stood at the counter. Any port in a storm.

"Hi, Dr. Henry."

He didn't look up from writing in a chart.

I waited.

Finally, he looked up. "Hi." That was all. He looked back at the chart.

In that brief "Hi," I saw his eyes. They were swimming pool blue, but blank. What was inside? It was worth another try. I held out the pack of newly purchased gum. "Would you like some gum, Dr. Henry?"

His head shot up, the blue eyes piercing. "It had better be sugar-free gum! You can't have regular gum."

I felt as if he had slapped me. Hard. My hand fell away, pulling back the potentially criminal gum.

His blue eyes glared.

I stared back, and he returned to the hospital chart. I stepped back, holding my gaze. What had just happened? He was a terrifying mystery that snapped out and stung like a wasp.

I turned slowly and walked on eggshells toward the ward. What a day. I had witnessed that the claws of sickness shred at their own will, but I could fool the world by pushing up the corners of my mouth...I could turn into a robot and hide my heart in a deep frozen place...I had reveled in my Grandiose Event, been devastated by its end, and stung by a scorpion disguised as a doctor.

In the ward, a naked iron bed sat where Theresa used to be. I wondered how she was doing in ICU. Was she white as a ghost like Susi, connected to a thousand tubes, moaning and throwing up green foam? Would anyone hold her hand and stroke her face when she was afraid? She was so calm about everything....had she turned to a robot, too?

I imagined being flipped like a pancake from my stomach to my back every hour. How scary. What if they dropped her? How did they manage to keep all the tubes straight when they flipped her? What if her IV came out during flipping, and they had to stick and gouge her all over again? My head ached.

I put on my pink gown and got into bed. Closing my eyes, I hoped that sleep would come quickly. I listened for Susi's cry, but fortunately only quiet snores came from her bed. Maybe tomorrow would be more normal...whatever that was.

Lessons Learned:

1. There are a lot of horrible things in the world - diabetes might not be the worst.
2. With tremendous thinking and effort, I can keep myself from barfing.
3. Maddie is a magician, and making me beautiful on the outside heals parts of my insides.
4. Planning can keep everything in control, but only some of the time.
5. Grandiose Events are wonderful on the uphill side, but very hard on the downhill.
6. Cousin Tommy has turned into a *man*, and said I am gorgeous. How very, very odd.
7. People who go to medical school may come out in strange non-human form.

CHAPTER 8

I awoke realizing it was President's Day. At home my classmates were out of school, but school at the hospital would happen. I made up my mind - today was my own personal holiday. After all, did I not share a birthday with Abraham Lincoln? I did indeed.

Activity in the ward did not allow for more sleep. Nurses zoomed in and out, breakfast trays slapped onto tables, roommates stumbled out of bed and turned on lights. I lay quietly, studying the activity...a veritable anthill.

Veritable is a good strong word. It leaves no doubt to the reality of a thing, no room for question. It literally stresses the aptness of a metaphor. In fact, that is part of the definition, so I am being redundant. It's good to have personal holidays so you can think about things like this.

"Hey, Rachel, you better get up, or you'll be late for school!" It was Patricia.

"I'm not going to school, it's a holiday."

"There are no holidays here. You can't not go."

"Yeah? Just watch." I sat on the edge of the bed, putting on my pink slippers and robe in slow motion, like a Kung Fu movie. Oozing drama, I sauntered to the bathroom door, turning to Patricia to give a Miss America smile and wave.

She grinned. "You're gonna get in trouble."

"Really? What can they do to me they haven't already? Strip me naked? Nope, too late for that. Stab me with needles? Oops, already done that, too! You know what? I think the only thing left is physical torture, and it's against the law." I sniffed haughtily.

"You're nuts! They'll probably come with a gurney, tie you down and wheel you to school!"

"Them and whose army?" I yanked open the bathroom door, slammed it behind me, and turned the lock.

"Okay, I'll cover for you. I'll tell Mrs. Bradshaw you died."

We fell into fits of laughter. I heard her steps tap out the door and recede down the hallway. I was now alone. I did not feel quite so gutsy. I collected pee in the steel pitcher, and took a shower. Just because I wasn't going to school didn't mean I planned to be dirty all day. Back at my bed, I pulled the privacy curtain and got dressed. Instead of opening the curtain, I let its safety hold me. What would happen next? Would a nurse come in and yell at me? If so, what would I say? Dread bounced on a trampoline inside my stomach.

I sat on the bed and waited, but not for long. Under the curtain I saw white nurse shoes walk into the ward, hesitate, and approach my bed. A nurse I didn't know broke through my haven of refuge.

"Aren't you supposed to be in school?" The nurse had red hair and freckles, and looked like she was about Mom's age. She wore a pointy white cap that resembled a tiny witch's hat.

"No, it's President's Day. That's a holiday, you know."

She looked confused. "That doesn't matter. You still have school here."

Dread did a back-flip, but my moment of liberation had come. "I'll not be attending school today." My voice was steady.

"Now, look, you can't just hang around here all day doing nothing. You have to go to school. If you don't go, I'll get one of the doctors."

Sitting cross-legged on my bed, I looked straight into her green eyes and said, "I'll not be attending school today." I turned away and poked through the over bed table for my reading book. When I glanced back, she was still there.

I ignored her gaze and opened the Hardy Boys. Joe Hardy was telling Frank about the mysterious visitor he had before finding a dead body in the garden. As the Hardy brothers ran toward the garden, I looked up again.

She was gone.

Relief. I returned to the Hardy Boys. Just as the boys tripped over the dead body, I heard paired footsteps approaching. Apparently Witch Hat had gone for reinforcements. The curtain around my bed was snatched open, completely invading my holiday.

"What's going on here?" One of the residents stood in front of me. He looked about Tommy's age, with sandy blond hair and blue eyes, like I imagined Joe Hardy.

"I'm not going to school today." My heart raced, but my voice held. I kept thinking, *You can lead a horse to water, but you can't make her drink.*

"Why do you think you're not going to school?" The resident was trying to sound authoritative. It wasn't working. He sounded more curious than adamant.

"You people seem very opinionated about school."

"Opinionated?" He smiled. "That's a pretty big word for a little girl. Don't' you want to learn more big words like that at school?"

I explained about Presidents' Day.

He looked at the floor for a moment. His eyes came back to mine. "What will you do around here all day? Won't you get bored?"

"I rarely get bored."

His smile broadened. "Well, if you do, you can always go to the schoolroom. Otherwise, have a nice holiday."

Witch Hat whipped a scowl his direction.

Oblivious, he walked toward the door. Witch Hat marched after him snorting tendrils of steam.

I stretched out on my bed, spreading the Hardy Boys over my face. Time for a Victory Nap.

"Wow! I can't believe you're still here." Patricia trotted into the ward, and woke me up. It was morning break, my Victory Nap was over.

"Yeah, I actually *won.* Can you believe it?"

She looked at me with the kind of awe I had seen on TV shows, when a single cowboy outwitted an entire posse, several tribes of Indians, bounty hunters and Matt Dillon. "Think we should all do the same thing, and skip out this afternoon?"

"Uh...you'll have to decide for yourself." I had not planned to set off a group mutiny.

Jenny strolled in. "Mrs. Bradshaw wanted to know where you were. We told her you were having a holiday, and you know what? I don't think she even cared! I don't get it."

We looked quizzically at each other. I thought bucking the system would be harder than this. Something told me to remember today, because system bucking would be required again.

In the meantime, I had things to do. I pulled out my new scrapbook and sack of Get Well cards from mail call. Mail from my friends and family was amazing - I got more than anyone else in the ward. Mom sent a note to our hometown paper about my diabetes, and included the hospital address. I had mail from people at church, my classmates, and folks I did not even know...apparently friends of Mom and Dad. Granny sent at least one card every day, sometimes two, and occasionally she enclosed cash. I had no need for money, but it was nice just in case. Knowing people at home recognized my plight as a big deal softened the harshness. This was the biggest life-or-death thing to happen to me personally. Dad's heart attacks when I was seven and eleven, and Janis' seizures from low blood sugar jarred my world, but they had not attacked my own personal body. This required a Memorial. Hence, the scrapbook.

I sorted through cards. Between Memorial building, the Hardy Boys, and pondering words, there was plenty to keep me busy through school hours. I chuckled, thinking about Joe-Hardy-resident believing I might get bored. He obviously did not comprehend the immensity of life.

"Oh crap!" Jenny stomped out of the bathroom shaking her test tube. It was orange-red. "Look at this! Not a little sugar, but four plus...and I've been doing all the stuff I'm supposed to."

I looked at her, and got a flashback of our earlier conversation.

She read my mind. "I *have*! I haven't squirted out my insulin. I've taken *every* stupid shot, and this is my thanks. Nothing works right with diabetes, it's all crap."

Her frustration soaked into me; I knew how she felt. "Hey, let's go run stairs! That'll help, won't it?"

Jenny scowled, pacing back and forth, shaking the orange-red test tube. "I guess...as if it'll do any good."

I hopped off the bed and pulled Jenny to the nurse's station. "Jenny and I are gonna run stairs. Her sugar is four plus."

One of the nurses looked up."Okay. Is your sugar high, too?" she directed at me.

"No. It's negative."

The nurse looked tentative. "Well, be careful. If you feel at all low, come immediately back to the floor." She handed me packets of soda crackers. "Take these in case of emergency, and don't get off on any other floors."

I thought how exceptionally weird it was to take a packet of soda crackers for an "emergency". In the past, an emergency was something that required stitches, a plaster cast or Mom, not soda crackers.

We jogged down six flights of stairs, then back up three. We ran down two more flights, and back up three. It became a vertical game of follow-the-leader, accompanied by loud giggling and yelling.

"I'm the leader now!" I yelled at Jenny, and dashed up the stairs. I missed a step and caught myself. For some reason I had double-vision. The stairway blurred and I felt suddenly exhausted.

Jenny passed me, running higher.

I held the railing for dear life, because the steps had gone into full spin.

"Hey, are you coming? I'm leading now," Jenny yelled from the landing above.

"Jenny....." I shook, and sweat poured down my face.

"You okay?" Jenny walked down toward me.

Looking up, I saw two of her. "I...don't...know." The words bounced around several times in my head before coming out.

"Eat your crackers, Rachel. Do it now!" Jenny tore open the packet and shoved crackers in my mouth.

"...mm...caa'n...eat. Mouf...dry." The crackers stuck to my tongue.

"Yes, you can. Eat 'em *now!*" She was suddenly the girl-in-charge.

I chewed, and finally a scratchy wad of cracker slid down my throat. "I'm sweating like crazy, but freezing. Is this a heart attack, like the doctors said?"

Jenny shot me a withering look. "No, dummy. You're having an insulin reaction. We've been running stairs for ten minutes, and you were negative when we started. You're paying for my high sugar."

I sat in silence and churned my crackers. "Whaddya mean, I'm paying for your high sugar?"

"When your blood sugar is low, you can't run around without eating something. It's nice of you to run stairs with me, but you gotta be prepared. You won't live long with diabetes if you're not."

I was getting lectured from a girl who skipped her insulin shots. The sweating stopped, but I was clammy as a fish. "Jenny, I'm freezing. What's the deal?"

"That's how it is: you get shaky, sweaty and weak. When you start to come out of it you get freezing cold, and can't warm up."

She was right. The cold came from somewhere deep inside me. "What if these crackers aren't enough?"

Jenny's eyes locked on mine. "I'll get help if you need it; keep chewing."

Time passed: a second or a day? Something inside me began to regroup. It all pulled together quickly like I was being sucked out of a black hole, but the sweat-soaked clothing remained as proof. I stood up. I wanted to get back to the nurse's station before it happened again.

"We're not walking up any more stairs. We're taking the elevator."

"We can't. The nurse said not to get off on other floors."

"Yeah? Well, the nurse can eat dirt." Jenny helped me up and pulled me through the stairwell door.

"How will we find the elevator?"

"All these floors look the same, they're just painted different colors."

"How do you know?"

"I run these stairs all the time, except usually I do it alone. I like to explore."

"So, you've gotten off on the wrong floor before?"

She shot the withering look again. "*Wrong* floor? It's *a* floor."

"But the nurse said..."

"Where are you *from*?! Do you follow every stupid rule somebody puts in front of you? How do you ever *learn* anything?"

"Hey! If you remember, it was *me* who decided not to go to school on President's Day, and you just went right along with the rules. Here's the deal...when rules make sense, I follow 'em. When they don't, I figure out what does."

Jenny strode on saying nothing; I marched along beside her. She was right about the floors, this one looked exactly like ours, except blue instead of green. Everything was blue: floor tiles, walls, even the ceiling. We reached the elevator and Jenny pushed the button.

"I'd take us down to the lobby for a look around, if you weren't low."

I was in awe of Jenny's independence, but afraid for her at the same time.

The elevator screeched, and opened.

Jenny herded me inside. "I do the same as you."

"What?"

"I follow the rules that make sense to me, but with diabetes there are too many to make sense. Everybody has a set of rules to lay on you - my doctor has a set, my mom has another, Dad has his rules, when I come to the clinic or hospital and see that whole herd of doctors, they all have a different set, too. The only rule that's the same for all of them is, 'Do what I say or you'll die of diabetes.' I think that's crap, so I make my own as I go."

The elevator squealed to a stop. "What if your rules aren't right?"

"Then I'll figure out something else. If all I hear from doctors and my mom is how diabetes is gonna wreck me, forget it. What's the point?"

A prickly ball swelled in my stomach. "Yeah, but I don't want to die of diabetes. I don't want to go blind. I don't want to have my legs sawed off, but I want to be able to go bare-foot. I don't want to have a stroke or heart attack. I don't want to live on a dialysis machine....whatever that is. I'm going to try to do all the stuff they say, and hope they're right."

"What if they're not? What if you do all that, and still go down the tubes?"

"I dunno."

"Good luck. Maybe we'll live to be as old as our parents, maybe we won't."

I started laughing. "Geez, living that long should be long enough for *anybody!*"

We had a giggling fit. Leaning against the concrete wall, we slid to the floor gasping for air. As old as our parents...omigosh!

Lessons Learned:
1. Standing your ground is very important. Life calls for a lot of it.
2. Something as simple as playing with a friend can suck you into the Neverland of low blood sugar. Those unprepared will never come back.
3. Rules are for the faint of heart; survivors hack a path through the jungle. (Will I make it through the jungle?)

CHAPTER 9

The day finally came: I was going home. Though it was the hope of my every waking hour for the past two-and-a-half weeks, now I was scared to death. What if my tests turned orange? The responsibility of diabetes control was moving from the hospital staff shoulders to mine, and the weight was crushing.

I knew how to decrease my insulin over the next several weeks for what the doctors called my "honeymoon phase". That meant my pancreas temporarily recovered. It could last from days to months, but what if my pancreas eloped? What if I failed at being *diabetic*? My brain went into a death spiral. Sometimes being a thinker is way too hard.

"Ready to go, punkin?" Daddy strode into the ward with his usual air of ownership. He saw my face, "Hey, you okay?"

"Daddy, what if I die?" Tears gathered.

"Whoa!" He rushed to my side, knelt down, and put his arms around me.

Panic wavered.

"We can deal with this. Remember, all the stuff we've learned?"

"Will you help me?" A tear made its way down my left cheek.

Daddy whipped out the ever-ready handkerchief and captured it with a soft wipe. "We can do this. Mostly, you'll do it, because you're with it twenty-four hours every day, but I'll back you up."

Even diabetes couldn't mess with Dad. I snuggled into his arms, and the fear disappeared. In its place grew a wild weed of Confidence.

"Okay then, here's the plan. The nurse has ordered insulin, syringes, a tester kit, extra pills and test tubes, as well as a gram scale for me. We have to go down to the storeroom in the basement floor to pick them up. She told me where it is. As soon as we get all that stuff and check back at the nurse's station, we can go home. I'm packed, c'mon." I jerked him toward the door with new superhuman strength.

"Uh...okay." Dad stumbled, then fell into step beside me. We headed to the elevator. In the storeroom I collected and checked off each item.

"It's all here, Dad. Can you carry the sacks?" I motioned toward the mound of equipment on the counter.

He picked up our booty, and staggered behind me.

Back in the ward, I packed supplies. Then I stripped my hospital bed, as an act of finality.

"We're ready."

"You sure?" He double checked my vacant locker. "Anybody you want to tell good-bye?"

"Nope. Jenny and Patricia went home days ago. I said goodbye to Maddie last night on evening shift, and Mrs. Bradshaw when I got my schoolbooks." Even little Susi had miraculously recovered and went home a week ago. I always wondered what had made her so sick...besides the surgery, I mean. Theresa never returned to the ward. As far as I knew she was still flipping like a pancake every hour in the ICU. The thought made me shudder, but this was my day - I was the last refugee out of camp.

"Let's go! You pull the car around. I'll wheel stuff down." I was in high gear. Speeding from the ward, I rounded the corner to the nurse's station with Dad in hot pursuit. "We're checking out," I bull-horned at a pointy white cap behind the nurse's station.

A red headed nurse looked up. It was Witch Hat. "Oh...?"

Dad took over. "Rachel and I are ready to check out. We've gotten her equipment." He was ready to make a break for it, too.

"Let me make a final check on your equipment." Witch Hat took far too long itemizing every bag. Finally she was satisfied. "Okay, Mr. Gifford, it looks like you have everything. Take care." She looked down at me, "Be sure you go to school when it's not a holiday."

"What?" Dad looked at her quizzically.

"C'mon Dad, we need to get on the road." I barreled down the hallway.

Finally in the car, Dad headed up highway sixty-three, and my brain slowed from a gallop to a trot. As telephone poles flew by, peace tip-toed into my heart. Even the cloudy brownness of an early March countryside cast no gloom.

That lasted until Kirksville, forty-five minutes from home. As we drove through town I saw the college, and places our family had gone for dinner or a movie. I shivered. I was not the same girl I had been then, and I never would be her again. Today, blindness lurked around every corner. Spring would no longer see me barefoot in new grass. Kidney disease and dialysis hovered as a sword of Damocles.

What if Jenny was right? What if the doctors did not have all the answers? What if, regardless of what I did, my diabetes screwed up? I shut my eyes to barricade threatening tears, but it was no use.

Why, God? Why? The words echoed in my head. *Okay, here's the deal. I don't know why You gave me this disease, but...I will do everything in my power to take care of myself, if You will let me be healthy and live long enough to see why You gave it to me.* He heard it. The ball was in His court now.

Car wheels crunched in the driveway - we were home. Our house looked the same: tall, two-story Victorian, pale yellow siding with white trim, and screen doors with a "G" on the scrollwork. The yellow siding and screen doors came two years ago when Dad had a great winter wheat crop, and the market went up. Otherwise, money for the house, and everything else for that matter, took second place to what we owed the hospital and clinic. Between Dad's heart attacks, Janis' diabetes, and now my diabetes, second place was usually no place.

Dad unloaded my stuff. As we hauled it into the house I felt like an alien from Mars. In the last two-and-a-half weeks I had changed from a little girl to a young adult. How does an adult act in the house of her youth?

We walked up the stairs to the porch that wrapped the front half of the house. Holly and I had ridden tricycles around that porch for hours at a time. Janis had jumped her pogo stick up and down the steps, and out to the sidewalk landing, that spread eight feet across the width of the stairs. Though a thinker, I lacked the balance and guts required to be a pogo-er.

I remembered the Easter all three of us kids were ready for church, and waiting for Mom and Dad on the porch. Janis got bored and grabbed her pogo stick. It was an amazing sight. She wore a white dress shimmering with silver threads, her first pair of nylons and pumps, and a white hat that matched her shoes. She bounded across the yard pogo-ing high in the air as her hat flew off, landing in Mom's flowerbed. Janis never looked back. She pogo-ed halfway down the block before careening into a neighbor's mail box. Regrouping in the road, she pogo-ed the rest of the block to the high school before Mom and Dad came outside. Holly and I were enraptured!

When Mom and Dad arrived, they were less enthusiastic. Janis pogo-ed home pronto, grabbed her hat from the flowerbed, and slapped it on as we sped off to church. She was the Pogo Queen.

It was a good memory to hold as I walked into the kitchen.

"Nancy, we're home!" Dad dropped my suitcase by the door as Mom burst in from her sewing room.

"Giff! Rachel! You're *home!* Oh, I'm *so glad!* Give me a hug!" Mom encompassed me.

I hugged her back, wondering if she could feel that part of me had not made it home. "Look Mom, I have all my equipment. I need to get it put away, and eat my snack, because it's almost three o'clock."

"Okay." Mom looked at my boxes. "Do you want help?"

"No, I can do it. Where should I store the food scale?"

"Um...maybe by the stove?"

I zeroed the scale, and checked my meal plan for the afternoon snack: one fruit and one milk exchange. It was two-thirty, so there was time to unpack. Hauling my suitcase upstairs, I dragged it onto my bed and surveyed the room. Janis was not around, but it was obvious she had cleaned our room for my homecoming. Usually her clothes decorated surfaces of furniture, as well as the floor. Janis felt hanging up clothes and putting things away was a limitation of her personal Bill of Rights. Her Rights often found their way across the border to my territory, limiting my Right to be tidy. Such was the life of two sisters.

I headed back downstairs for the rest of my equipment, and met Dad coming up with his arms full.

"Hey, punkin', don't you need some help with this stuff?"

"Thanks, Dad!" Dad understood about getting organized. He and Mom had the same feeling about organization that Janis and I did about tidiness. Opposites attract. It was a loud point of contention in our household.

He deposited the tonnage on my desk. "Need help unpacking?"

"No, Dad. This is my job; I can take care of it."

He gave me a wink. "I know you can, kiddo. Nobody can do it better than you." He patted my back and headed down.

I hoped he was right.

The urine tester went on my cupboard shelf in the bathroom. Each of us kids had our own shelf. Often, Janis or Holly would put their things on other shelves, or in completely uncharted destinations, and lose them. This made no sense to me. If the time they spent looking for things was totaled cumulatively it might add up to weeks. Why would anyone want to spend weeks of their life looking for things if they had a shelf? It probably tied back to the personal Bill of Rights.

I checked my watch: two-forty. It would take ten minutes to weigh and measure my snack, so I had ten minutes left to unpack. Undies went in the second-to-top bureau drawer, dresses, slacks and blouses hung in the closet, dirty clothes went in the pink hamper in the corner. The hamper was stuffed full of Janis' clothes. Clean-room-mystery - solved.

My laundry went on top of the hamper; I would take them to the washer when I went to fix my snack. Almost done at twelve minutes to three. The last sack of supplies contained syringes, alcohol wipes, insulin, mixing bottles and extra tablets for my urine tester. Where on earth would I put all this stuff?

I checked my top bureau drawer. This had always been my Treasure Drawer. It was full of amazing and magical things: nearly empty make up jars and tubes handed down from Mom and Janis, plastic rings from gum ball machines, toys from Cracker Jacks (which I could never eat again), ribbons, small stuffed animals, things I had made in Bible School, glitter, glue, scraps of paper with pictures I had drawn...wonderful things. I sighed. They were useless really, child's toys. I pulled out the drawer and dumped the contents in the trashcan. Treasures were replaced by diabetes supplies.

My feet were heavy as I plodded toward the kitchen. I measured my snack and ate without tasting.

"What time is dinner, Mom?"

"I'm not sure. Are you still hungry?" Mom looked perplexed.

"No. Even if I was I can't eat anything else until dinner." I would think she knew that after taking care of Janis for so long. I would be wrong.

"I need forty minutes warning so I can test and get my shot. I can help you set the table after that." I put my dishes into the sink.

"Do you need help with any of this?" Her look said she was trying to figure me out.

"Nope. This is my disease. No one can handle it but me. When you get ready to make a shopping list, let me know, because I need to be sure we get fresh fruit, fruit canned without sugar, green beans and skim milk. Also lunchmeat for school lunches, graham crackers, and Vanilla Wafers. Vanilla Wafers are an allowed treat, counted as both bread and fruit exchanges. When I go to Granny's we'll have to be sure I have my sugar-free canned fruit, because Granny will have the kind in syrup."

Mom looked dazed. "Okayyy...do you need help with your shots?"

I dreaded this question. Shots in my thighs or abdomen were no problem, but when it came to my hip or arm it was harder. Regardless, I did not want to have Mom give my shots. It hurt more when the nurses injected me, and I was afraid it would be the same with Mom. I also knew Mom liked to try new injection sites with Janis. She had given Janis a shot in the back of her shoulder once, and Janis moaned for a half hour afterward. I did not want to be Mom's experiment.

"You know, Mom, I was thinking maybe Janis could help me. Since we're both diabetic, we know what shots feel like." I gave her my in-control smile.

"Okay, I think Janis will like that."

I breathed a quiet sigh.

"We don't need to go to all that bother with the sugar free canned fruit. It's so expensive. I have regular canned fruit that we can use if we just pour off the syrup and rinse." Mom gave me her in-control smile.

I had two-and-a-half weeks of diabetes training under my belt, and in all that time nobody had talked about pouring syrup off canned fruit. What if it made my blood sugar go up? "I only know one way to control my diabetes, and it calls for fruit that is fresh, dried, or canned in water or juice."

"That's childish silliness! I have a degree in Home Economics, and I certainly know about food."

"I have to deal with what I know."

Mom looked at the floor; I think she counted to ten. "Have it your way, but specially canned fruits cost good money." She was pulling out the trump card. Money was always the final answer.

"If you don't have the money, it could come out of my allowance."

"You just *have* to have things your way!"

"Thanks." I didn't wait for further reply; I was upstairs before she could take another breath. Back in my room I recouped. Mom was probably right, but if she wasn't, I would be the loser, not her. I shuddered. Sometimes we had such a hard time with each other.

"Forty minutes before supper's on," Mom hollered up the stairs.

Time had slipped by while I rechecked my food exchange booklet for the errant syrup-canned-but-rinsed-fruit. It just wasn't in there. I hurried to the bathroom, collected my urine specimen and did my test. The concoction boiled. Some improvements had been made in the test kit since Janis got hers. My kit required only one pill, and it boiled by a chemical reaction instead of actual fire. It also took less time. I watched the navy blue color appear and felt myself relax. Then it turned green. I caught my breath. I shook the tube and compared it to the color chart. It was between trace and one percent.

"No!" I ran downstairs shaking the tube in front of me.

Mom came running from the kitchen. "What's wrong?"

"It's green, I'm almost one percent. This never happened at the hospital!" I put the test tube in the kitchen sink and sank onto a chair. Nausea churned in my stomach.

"You're overreacting. You rode in the car all day so you had less activity, that's why you have a little sugar." She held up the test tube. It didn't look quite as threatening in her hands. "It's not even one percent, it's barely trace. It'll be back down by tomorrow. If not, we can go up on your insulin."

She was right. I tried to breathe normally. Closing my eyes, I imagined, no *willed*, my bedtime test to turn blue.

I took my shot and measured my food, leaving out a bread exchange. Maybe it would help bring down my sugar. I kept this decision to myself.

Ten thirty p.m. - I watched the concoction boil in my test tube. It turned blue, then fell silent. A sob of relief caught in my throat. Somewhere inside my head I realized the absurdity of my immense relief, and wondered if I would be this absurd the rest of my life.

Lessons Learned:
1. Going home from the hospital is a blessing, and a curse.
2. Responsibility for your own life or death is a heavy weight.
3. I went to the hospital a little girl, but I came home a very old and nervous adult.
4. The only thing harder than accepting my disease, is trying to wrench it from Mom.

CHAPTER 10

Monday morning came a half hour earlier than it had on school days before diabetes. It would take that long to do my test, take my shot, weigh and measure my breakfast, as well as my ten a.m. snack and lunch, and get all the food and equipment packed. My planning and preparation equaled that of the Boston Tea Party.

At school I would put my snack in my desk. When the other kids went for morning break I would chug my milk and snarf down my graham crackers, then catch up with them. No one would be the wiser.

I still had to figure out how to test my urine without being conspicuous in the girls' bathroom. I needed to combine water from the faucet, with urine. I did not want to gross out people by taking a cup of pee to the sink. After testing, how could I dump the cup of pee in the toilet, go back to the sink for water to rinse the cup, back to the toilet to dump that, without being a pariah?

I closed my eyes and pictured the stall inside the girls' restroom. I had it! Before I peed, I could use the dropper to get clean water from the toilet bowl, putting drops in the test tube. I would catch my urine in the cup and do the test. When it was done, I would empty the cup and test into the toilet, and flush. When clean water came into the bowl I would rinse the test tube and cup, then dry the kit with toilet paper. It was gross, but I would wash my hands really well afterward.

It would take a long time in the stall, so I needed to do it when the bathroom was less crowded. Maybe if I went directly to the restroom before lunch, everyone else would be in the lunchroom. That would make me late for lunch, but while my class waited in the cafeteria line, I would sit down and brown-bag it. It could work.

I thought about this school year. Sixth grade had been filled with both light and shadow. I was thrilled finding out Mrs. Barker would be my teacher. She was a beautiful lady who loved children. I knew this, because love beamed from her face when she smiled at us. She wore glasses that hung from a delicate beaded necklace when they were not on her nose. She looked up from her work when any of us walked in the classroom, and always greeted us like we had done something special.

The shadow of sixth grade was that I lost my best friend. As small children, Molly (whose real name is even prettier) and I lived across a gravel country road from each other. After our families moved to town for school, we had been in the same classroom every year since kindergarten. We called each other on the phone, and talked in the evening. This year things had changed. Molly was not in Mrs. Barker's class. I was sorrier about that than I could express.

I consoled myself by thinking we would still see each other at lunch and recess. I was wrong. Molly found a new group of friends, and I was not in it. My heart free-fell into a pit. I worked at making new friends in sixth grade, but new friends are not the same as old friends. Going back to school with diabetes would have been easier if I still had a best friend.

As I stood pensively on the porch with Holly, waiting for the bus, Janis walked to the high school building only a block from our house. My test kit and food were packed carefully inside my school bag. Only I would know all the thought, preparation and planning that went into looking normal. I hoped.

Things went according to plan up to morning break: The first opportunity for Exposure. All my classmates hurried out for break; I lingered behind, shuffling through papers and slowly putting books into my desk. I wished Mrs. Barker would leave like the rest of the class so I could snarf down my food and get on with trying to fit in.

"How are you feeling? You look wonderful!" Mrs. Barker gave me her sunshine smile as she walked toward me.

I smiled back. "Oh, fine. Thank you. Just fine. I'm really glad to be out of the hospital." I was nervous. I did not want to talk about the hospital, so why had I brought it up?

"We're very glad to have you back."

"Thank you."

"Don't you want to take a break?"

I could see I would have to tell her I needed to eat a snack. Food was prohibited in the schoolroom, but I hoped and prayed she would make an allowance. I cleared my throat. "Mrs. Barker, as part of my diet I have to eat a small snack at ten o'clock. It's in my desk, and I need to eat it now, before all the kids come back and ask a lot of questions." I pulled the graham crackers and warm milk out of my desk.

"Oh my...we're not supposed to allow food in the classroom." Now Mrs. Barker looked nervous.

"I have only ten minutes to eat my snack and take a bathroom break. Please don't make me go somewhere else to eat. I'll be late for class." My voice was pleading. I had not meant to plead. I shoved graham crackers in my mouth like a starving pig.

"Well, I guess maybe we can make an exception for today. I'll check with the Principal to find out how to do this in the future." She wanted to help me, but now my diabetes was causing trouble for her, too. This *stupid* disease! It caused trouble for everyone.

I washed down the ball of graham crackers with lukewarm milk. It tasted pretty bad, but it was done. "Thank you. Thank you for understanding. It will be easier if we can keep this as low key as possible. I don't want to look like I'm getting special privileges or doing things other kids don't. It'll just make things harder." I was babbling.

Mrs. Barker hesitated. "Has that glass of milk been in your desk all morning? It must be warm!"

"Um....yes. But that's okay."

Her eyes looked sad and worried. "Rachel, you can't drink warm milk. It must taste terrible!"

"No, Mrs. Barker. No, it's okay. Please excuse me, so I can use the restroom before the bell rings for class." I dashed out the door, leaving her to her own thoughts. My time was limited; one hurdle down, several more to go.

The bell blared for lunch, the signal for my urine test. I had mentally rehearsed my plan several times. Making a bee-line for my locker, I grabbed the test kit. "Rachel! Want me to save you a place in the lunchroom?"

Susan, my locker-mate, called as I speed-walked (no running in the halls) toward the bathroom.

"That would be great! I'll look for you. I need to go get my lunch from the fridge."

"Okay, see you in a minute."

I knew it would be longer than a minute, but at least Susan was saving me a spot. So far, so good. I reached the bathroom and burst through the door: no one in sight. I went to the farthest stall and closed the door. I collected ten drops of water from the toilet bowl, put them in the test tube, and then peed in the cup.

The bathroom door opened and I heard loud voices. Who were they? Everyone was supposed to be at lunch! Now I would have to hurry. Five drops of urine, then the pill. There was no rushing this, the pill had to boil until it was done. Hours passed.

Finally the boiling stopped, and the mixture was blue. Yay! I dumped the urine and test, and flushed. Even the flushing took forever. I rinsed everything, and dried it with toilet paper.

"Who's in that end stall? Are they ever coming out? Geez!"

I heard group laughter. My face got hot. I tried to hurry faster, and dropped the cup. I recognized one of the voices; these were eighth grade girls! Oh why, oh why? I grabbed the cup just before it rolled under the toilet door. Now I *had* to stay in the toilet until they were gone; I couldn't walk out and face them. My plan faltered.

I packed my test kit and tried to get calm. They were at the sink washing their hands. I wondered if my class had finished eating and was ready to start lessons again. I looked at my watch. Only ten minutes had passed since I spoke with Susan. Relief! I was sure it had been several days.

I sat on the toilet and waited for the voices to leave. I remembered Dr. Jackson saying if my urine was negative for a week, I wouldn't need to test regularly at lunch anymore. The thought was calming. I imagined the girls giggling as they walked down the hall, talking about the weirdo camping out in the far stall, but they would never know who it was. Unless they recognized my shoes! Mental note: wear my Sunday shoes to school for three months until the heat dies down.

The voices were gone now. I walked out of the stall, free at last. I had made it with only one small falter. I was giddy. I giggled nervously all the way to my locker, put my test kit away, and was still giggling when I sat down by Susan.

"What's so funny?"

"Oh....just stuff. So whaddya have for lunch?" I looked at her plate. The only thing left was a remnant of meat loaf.

"Gross meat loaf. Yech! Whadda you have?"

. "Uh...bologna sandwich, milk and an apple." What I almost said was, "Two bread exchanges, two meat exchanges, a fruit, fat and milk exchange," but stopped myself just in time.

"Well, that's sure better than meat loaf. I wish my mom would pack my lunch. Then I could choose what I want instead of eating just whatever."

I gawked at Susan. "You'd rather carry your lunch than have hot lunch? Are you kidding?"

"Wouldn't you? Isn't that why you brought your lunch?"

"Uh...not exactly. I have to eat certain stuff since I got diabetes. I'd really rather have hot lunch."

"Oh. Maybe if I got diabetes my mom would pack my lunch."

I stared at Susan. There was not enough time in the universe to explain to her what an insane thing she just said. "Well, maybe you could pack your own lunch if you really want to bring it." I swallowed a hunk of bologna, realizing lunchtime was almost over.

"Pack my *own* lunch? Wow. I never thought of that. Do you pack your own lunch?"

It was hard to talk around the bologna. "Shurr...I even tell Mom what to buy for me at the grocery store. Sometimes I make a list, or go with her to be sure she gets the right stuff."

"*Really?* You *tell* your mom what to get for you?"

"How else would she know?" I was talking around bites of apple, and hoped I didn't spray her. I need not have worried. The look on her face said she was so amazed, a small cow could have been sitting in my lap, and it would not have registered.

The lunchroom was clearing, but I decided a few moments of conversation to enlighten Susan on how to handle getting what she needed, was an acceptable addition to my schedule. "Look, it isn't that hard. You just decide what you want to eat for the week, make a list, and ask your mom really nicely to get it for you when she goes to the grocery store. Offer to fix your own lunches, and if she doesn't like the idea, tell her it's cheaper than hot lunch. That'll cinch it."

"You're right! If I tell her it's cheaper, that's it." Susan stood up beaming with confidence. "Next week, I'm going to pack my lunch and bring what I want to school. No more stupid meat loaf!"

I shoved my lunch utensils into the paper sack, barely able to believe my good fortune. I would now have a comrade eating cold lunch with me, and she thought it was cool. Life had just gotten easier.

"Rachel, could I speak with you a moment?" Mrs. Barker caught me as Susan and I left the lunchroom.

My heart skipped a beat. What if she said I would have to leave class to eat my ten o'clock snack? "Yes, ma'am."

"I spoke with the Principal, and she said it would be all right for you to eat your snack at your desk. She felt it would be less disruptive than if you left class."

"Great! I mean thank you...I mean that's really great."

Mrs. Barker smiled and patted my shoulder.

I hopped off the school bus and ran toward the house. Holly and I did kangaroo jumps up each stair, reached the porch, and raced to the front door. The first day was over. It had to get easier from here.

I ran to the kitchen to fix my three o'clock snack. Holly beat me there and made a triple layer grape jelly sandwich. He wolfed it down and drowned it with a glass of milk. I weighed my sugar free pear half and measured a half cup of skim milk.

Holly watched. "Will you always have to do that?"

I kept my eyes on the measuring cup as skim milk poured from the carton. "Yeah, I think so."

Holly shook his head. "Seems like a pain to me."

"It's more than a pain. It's ridiculous, that's what it is! I felt like a total freak today!" The milk slopped across the counter as I yelled. I slammed the carton on the counter, and wiped up spilled milk. "But...it's how I stay alive now." I put the milk away and sat down.

Before diabetes, Holly and I were euphoric after getting off the bus. I usually had a triple layer grape jelly sandwich or two with him. We would gobble them down accompanied by glasses of milk, and then dash into the living room to watch *Dark Shadows* on TV. It always scared us silly; it was wonderful. Things had changed.

"You know, I'm really sorry." Holly looked sad.

"Yeah, me, too." We ate in silence.

"Hey! Let's go watch *Dark Shadows*!" Holly jumped up, shoved what was left of the triple-decker sandwich in his mouth, downed his third glass of milk and ran for the living room.

I gave my milk a quick slurp, which both started and finished it. I downed the pear half in one bite and dashed after Holly. It had been three weeks since I'd seen *Dark Shadows*. Heaven only knew what Barnabas Collins was up to these days. We parked in front of the TV. It was good to know some things had not changed.

Lessons Learned:

1. Taking care of diabetes without exposing the grossness of it, requires planning rarely known to people not in the business of espionage.
2. Helping friends get what they need sometimes helps me get what I need.
3. Much of my world has changed. A little bit has not, and for that bit I am grateful.

CHAPTER 11

Three months had come and gone since my hospitalization. Spring had sprung: Mom's tulips were blooming in the back yard, grass was turning green. Last Friday school ended for summer vacation. Life was going on, whether I had diabetes or not.

Today Mom and Dad would take Janis and me to the Medical Center for our check up. For Janis, this had been a regular thing for many years, now I would accompany her. It was an all day affair, between the six-hour round trip, and long clinic wait. I was not sure how Janis felt, but I was glad to have a comrade.

I had religiously done my tests and recorded the results. With the exception of my first day home from the hospital, they were all negative. Things had settled into a fairly consistent pattern. My record sheets contained the Litany of Life with Diabetes for the last quarter. Surely no fault could be found that would put me back into the hospital.

On the way out of town we made a stop at Granny's to pick up a home made to-go lunch. This was a Granny tradition. She made sandwiches from thick slices of ham, roast beef or home made meatloaf garnished with crispy bacon and spicy ketchup. Often she included (what we considered) her world famous fried chicken. At church carry-in dinners, people had been known to fight over the last chicken leg. When she made lunch for us grandkids, there usually was a sibling scuffle over the wishbone, accompanied by loud debates about rightful ownership and who had it last.

Granny made sure we had fresh apples or bananas, home made biscuits, and the coup de gras was her delectable oatmeal scotchies. Just thinking about those cookies made my mouth water. In the last few months however, I had learned to politely say, no-thank-you when they were offered. It was painful.

"Wow! Look at all these chicken legs!" Janis pawed through the lunch basket like a treasure chest, as we neared snack time. She snatched a chicken leg and half a meatloaf sandwich, putting them on a sturdy paper plate. Granny always included tableware and linens in her lunches. She said only "people who don't know any better" would eat right out of the box. It went without saying we should know better.

Mom turned from the front seat and eyed Janis' plate. "You can have the chicken leg *or* the half sandwich for your snack. Not both." Janis put back the sandwich and passed the basket to me. She did not seem to mind following Mom's orders; their relationship worked.

I was glad I knew exactly what to eat for my snack, and would not have Mom's prying eyes on me. Since getting diabetes, I had learned a new appreciation for food. I had learned to eat salad without dressing. By the time I measured dressing in the tablespoon, then spread it over the salad, there was not enough to matter. Why spend the time and a whole fat exchange? I was not in a position to decide if these changes were bad or good, they just were. Making the changes took so much energy, little was left-over for judging.

I took the basket and looked for fresh fruit I knew would be there. My morning snack was one fruit, and there it was: a huge Red Delicious apple. I drew it out, shining it with one of Granny's napkins. It was almost too pretty to eat. Turning it around I let the morning sun catch the sheen.

I sniffed in the sweet, tangy aroma, and, behind my eyes, I saw the mother tree covered in white ruffled blossoms. Bees dipped into the moist flowers and buzzed to their hive to make oozing golden honey. I crunched into the apple. Tart juice ran over my tongue and made my cheeks pucker. I held it up and looked at it. The inside was white as snow. It made me think of Snow White and the Seven Dwarves. Each bite changed the shape of the fruit. Bite-by-bite my apple went from a round fat fruit to a long slender fruit with a waistline. If I ate slowly the meat turned golden brown, adding a bit more interest. By pacing munches and nibbles, I might be able to make this apple last all the way to the Medical Center. Could be a record.

"Dad, how long to the Med Center from here?"

"On this road, probably about thirty minutes. Why?"

Mom gave him a you're-driving-too-fast look.

"I'm going to make my apple last, so let me know every time we go five miles, okay?"

"Sure, starting now?"

"Riiiiiiiiiiiiiiight *now!*" I took a small bite and munched daintily.

I had finished my thirty-seven minute apple by the time we drove into the Medical Center complex. We parked in the lot and took the shuttle bus to the clinic. It was quite a production. The complex looked as big as ever, but it was brighter in the late morning sun of early June, than it had been in the pale gray days of February.

Mom and Dad maneuvered through the long circuitous hallways leading to the clinic. Antiseptic assaulted my nose, and the halls looked like something from an Alfred Hitchcock movie. I should be dropping bread crumbs to find my way out.

When we reached the clinic, people were everywhere: sitting on metal straight chairs or wheelchairs, standing up leaning against the hospital-green wall, sitting or laying on the floor that was tiled in hospital-gray.

"Angela Johnston!" The exclamation was made by a tall, skinny nurse wearing a starched white dress, entirely free of wrinkles. She must have driven to work either standing or naked. She wore white stockings, white spotless shoes, and her nurse's hat was pointy on top. I remembered the pointy hat from my hospitalization. It came to me that nice nurses on the ward had not worn hats at all; they thought hats were stupid. "Look at that nurse's hat." I whispered in Janis' ear.

"Looks like a witch to me." Janis didn't bother to lower her voice, and looked straight at the nurse. It was Janis' way to be straight to the point, and sometimes embarrassing. "Who do you think Angela Johnston is, and what does the witch plan to do with her?"

"Probably one of the patients, like us, and she plans to bake her in a child-sized oven. What d'ya think?"

"Sounds right to me." Janis continued to stare at the pointy-hatted nurse, as her voice carried across the room.

My face got hot. "Maybe you should lower your voice."

"What for? She looks mean to me. Maybe we should bake her in a witch-sized oven?" We broke into indiscrete giggling. Janis had a motto: *Do unto others before they do unto you.*

Mom gave us a disapproving look; Dad looked more curious than disapproving. Mom was the self-appointed Disapprover.

85

"Angela Johnston! Calling Angela Johnston! The doctor will see you now!" Witch-nurse continued to beckon, and finally a dark-haired girl who looked a little younger than me stood up. A woman I placed as her mother accompanied her, and they disappeared through a doorway, led by Witch-nurse.

"Prob'ly the last we see of *that* little girl!" Janis tossed my direction.

"Girls!" Mom hissed.

We giggled into our hands.

"Why do you think they call us *patients*?" Janis shot at me.

"Uh...don't know. Because we have to wait so long?"

"Well I don't feel patient about it, do you?"

"No, *im*-patients would be more like it.

"It's a stupid name for human beings who are forced, against their will, to wait interminably in a goldfish bowl."

Hours, if not days, passed before Witch-nurse finally called what resembled our names.

"James and Rochelle Gifford! The doctor will see you now!"

Janis passed me a wondering glance. "Come on *Rochelle*! The doctor will see you now!"

"After you, *James*, be my guest!" I bowed low and extended my hand to let her pass.

We lined up single file and marched in cadence over to Witch-nurse.

She seemed a bit surprised.

Mother looked disapproving, and a sly grin spread across Dad's face.

"Mom, you don't need to go in with us. We'll be just fine." Janis gave her a wave of dismissal.

I was pretty sure Mom preferred not to be associated with us at this point, anyway.

Janis looked up at Witch-nurse. "Well, let's GO! We're burning daylight!"

Witch-nurse gave a start, and made a quick bee-line down the hall. We marched militarily behind her.

"James, this is your exam room." Witch-nurse looked down at Janis.

"Do I really *look* like James to you?" Janis' palms were firmly planted on her hips.

"Ah...no, dear, you don't." Witch-nurse looked suddenly puzzled.

"Well, that's good, because I'm not. So if I'm not James, who do you suppose I am?"

"Well, I'm not sure. Do we have your name wrong?"

"I'm Rochelle, for Pete Sake! Geez!" She jabbed her finger at me. "*That* is James!" She stomped into the exam room.

"Oh." Witch-Nurse was clearly flustered at this point. "Well, then James, you'll be in the exam room next to Rochelle."

"No, ma'am, Rochelle and I need to stay together. It looks like your waiting room is full of patients, so we can just share a room. We're more comfortable that way." I followed Janis' path into the exam room and perched cross-legged on the exam table.

"Okay..." Witch-Nurse laid our charts on the desk, and pointed to hospital gowns on the table. "Put those on, and the doctor will be in shortly."

Janis rose from her chair, popped her arms through the holes in the gown and sat down. She was fully clothed with her pink button-down oxford shirt sleeves poking out the armholes, and her burgundy stretch pants protruding beneath.

"No, you need to remove your clothes before putting on the gown." Witch-nurse's voice was tense.

"Really! That seems a little uncivilized, don't you think?" Janis gave her a look of shock.

"Well...perhaps, but that's how it's done." Witch-nurse was wilting under Janis' gaze.

Even at sixteen years of age Janis was more than five foot seven-and-a half inches tall, and her sarcasm could scathe Godzilla. "Fine! Then get the doctor."

Witch-nurse faltered with the doorknob, bumped into the door, and finally exited with great haste. The door closed behind her.

"Janis, I can't believe you!"

"Okay, here's the deal. When the stupid medical students come in here, we'll correct our names to Janis and Rachel, and then you're going to be me and I'll be you. Got it?"

"Great idea!" I got serious, we had to get into character.

Quickly we undressed and got into our costumes (hospital gowns). There was a knock at the door, a pause, and it opened a crack.

"Hello?" A bespectacled face pushed through the crack. He didn't look much older than Tommy. I felt kind of sorry for him, but certainly not sorry enough to ruin our ruse. Adrenalin rushed through my veins as the curtain rose.

"Come on in. Who are you?" Janis was on the offensive.

The face was followed by a tall skinny body that finally stepped around the corner of the door. "I'm Lawrence...er...Dr. Lawrence Todd."

"Are you really a doctor or are you a med student?" Janis began her inquisition.

"Oh. Well, I'm actually a resident."

"So, you live here?"

"No, no. I mean I'm doing my residency. We almost live in the hospital, I guess. It's my second year out of medical school." He smiled at Janis.

Janis smiled sweetly back: a bad sign for him. She was reeling him in and warming up the frying pan. "Oh...thank you for explaining. Let me explain our names to you." (Here it came...). "In the lobby the nurse called us James and Rochelle. As you can clearly see, neither of us is James. The names are Janis and Rachel. I'm Rachel, and this is my sister, Janis. It will make us feel more comfortable to call you Lawrence." She smiled the sweet smile again.

Lawrence smiled and looked more at ease. He was taking the bait; the line and sinker were not far behind. "Oh...thank you." He picked up my chart and looked at Janis. "So, Rachel, how have your first three months of diabetes been?

And so it went. Throughout the history-taking and physical exams he addressed Janis as Rachel and me as Janis, and wrote all his information in the corresponding chart. It was a powerful scene of acting with nary a character falter between us. The interview drew to a close. An academy award was imminent.

(Janis: still smiling) "So, what will you do with all this information you've recorded?"

(Lawrence: smiling in lamb-to-slaughter sort of way) "Oh, this is your chart, and it's your permanent record with the hospital. I'll present the information to your doctor before he comes in to see you."

(Janis: still smiling) "Great! I guess we'll see you later."

Lawrence exits, curtain falls.

Janis muffled her face in her hands, and I dived into the pillow as our giggles exploded.

Without warning, the door opened and Dr. Jackson walked in with Lawrence. Janis and I struggled valiantly, but we could not reclaim character.

"Looks like quite a trick you two pulled on Dr. Todd." Dr. Jackson gazed sternly at us.

Janis caught composure first. "Yes, I think Lawrence might have mixed up our charts."

Lawrence turned crimson. Tiny wisps of smoke curled out his ears.

"Let's see your record sheets." Dr. Jackson put on his glasses.

We pulled out our records and handed them over.

It had been a respectable opening night.

Lessons Learned:

1. Going to the diabetes doctor is a ridiculous hassle, improved considerably by Granny's fine lunch.

2. Food is more than nutrition. It stimulates imagination and provides entertainment, as well as fulfillment to the senses.

3. Clinic waiting rooms are as incompatible to humans as zoo cages are to elephants.

4. A little trickstering can improve any vulgarity...and Janis is the Trickster Queen.

CHAPTER 12

As Janis and I basked in our Thespianism, Dr. Jackson discussed with Mom and Dad an "opportunity" for me to participate in research. He discussed this opportunity as one might convey information about a project of Nobel Laureate proportions. Some might have thought this research would bring joy to the masses and feed all the starving children of the world. I was not in that group.

This research project was not simple, like filling out a questionnaire or participating in a half hour interview. It required I be hospitalized (incarcerated) for a full week. Each morning a team of doctors and nurses would come into (invade) my room, stick IV needles into my arms (torture me), give me experimental drugs (I do not even have a word for this), and record results (document my demise). The discrepancy in our perceptions was obvious. I was filled with terror, and immediately declined the offer, with a small, but firm one word answer, "No." Mother intervened.

Dr. Jackson continued as though I had never opened my mouth. "This is an exciting research protocol. It could give us new information about how to treat diabetes, and whether or not children with diabetes might be able to use oral drugs to treat their disease, or if they'll always have to take insulin. I postulate that insulin always will be required, but it warrants more research."

My heart skipped a beat. Deep in my soul I knew it was a ruse. I would never be able to use pills instead of shots, and my job description in this project was Resident Guinea Pig. Mom and Dad were teachers, so I knew a little about the academic world. Academicians have to publish articles to keep their jobs, and they have to do research for something to publish. The hand-writing was on the wall.

"No, thank you, Dr. Jackson. I don't want to be part of the research." There I'd said it again. I hoped my galloping heart would slow.

"Oh now, dear! We can think on this. This is important research Dr. Jackson wants to do!" Mom had that look in her eye. It said she was embarrassed with my behavior and wanted me to act sweetly, and go along with things.

I was not sure which was stronger, my terror or fury. Probably fury, because the terror dissolved into it. "Mom, I'm sure about this."

"We'll talk about it and get back to Dr. Jackson." The Exorcist movie had not yet been created, but if it had I would have expected Mom's head to make several complete rotations while her eyes gleamed with a sinister light.

I crumpled on the closest chair.

Conversation ensued between Mom and Dr. Jackson, but I did not hear what was said. I was busy keeping my own head from going into orbit while Mom sold me down the river.

The office visit finally ended, and after the room cleared Janis and I dressed quietly. A lifetime had passed since our wonderful joke on Lawrence.

"Janis, what do you think about this research thing?"

"I don't know."

"You don't know?!" I gaped at her.

"Well, if Mom and Dad think its okay, you'll probably have to do it."

I searched her eyes. What was there? Sincerity...but something was missing. "Do you *get* what this *means*? I'll have to go back into the hospital again for a whole week. I'd rather die than do that. Do you get me? I'm not being dramatic here. I'd rather die."

Janis shrugged.

I had to fight this. I must make them have *my* interest at heart. Surely Dad would listen. I could get more logic from him than Mom. I thought of the three-hour car ride home, and decided that was when I would somehow make them see my point.

What was it with this damnable research? (There I went with bad words again.) Years before my diabetes was diagnosed, Mom had made Holly and me be part of a research study at the Medical center. It was supposed to tell if either of us might get diabetes later in life. Like I wanted to know?

Mom and Dad believed research was the answer to anything. Research and God, the answers to all questions known to humanity. They had willingly sacrificed Holly and me at the altar of science.

For the research we had to leave home at four o'clock in the morning to drive to the University Medical Center in Columbia to start the testing by seven-thirty a.m. Mom and Dad could eat breakfast, but Holly and I could not. We had to be "fasting", which is a medical term for starving-to-death. The researchers gave us a way-too-sweet lemonade drink that could rot your teeth on contact. We had to dump it into our way-too-empty-and-carsick stomachs, and then the researchers stabbed our fingers for blood samples several times every half hour for four hours. Only two good things came from this - my fingers were too sore to practice piano lessons for a week, and I got so sick from the lemonade that I threw up on the lady who stabbed our fingers.

My justice was short-lived however. The White Coat people declared I must complete the four hours of testing whether I threw up or not, *and* if my test values were not in the range they expected, I would have to return and start the test all over another day. At this point you would think any parent, caring about the betterment of their children, would have intervened. If you put my mom and dad in that category, you would be wrong. I ended up doing both.

When I complained about the unfairness of this ordeal Mom, too cheerfully, reminded me that I should simply be grateful that I did not have diabetes, and have to take shots the rest of my life. I wondered if diabetes might be easier. Now I knew, I was wrong. But *now*, even *having* this monster disease, she *still* was making me be a guinea pig!

Janis and I finished dressing and walked to the waiting room.

"There you are! We're ready to go." Mom was using her cheery voice. She patted my shoulder.

I stiffened and pulled away. She had turned into a plastic Mommy doll. If you pulled her string, out came Mommy chat and Mommy pats.

We would have been a fascinating study for a psychologist, as the four of us boarded the shuttle bus, and then walked to the car. Mom and Dad discussed the clinic visit, the upcoming trip home and where to eat dinner. Janis piped in from time to time with her opinion of where to eat, and I was silent as a stone. Was there anything underneath their chatter? Was I the only one who realized I was a dead-man-walking?

Four car doors slammed. Dinner was over, and my strategy had grown with every bite. I would wait until we were out of city traffic and safely on the long road home, then begin litigation.

City blocks flew by as we neared the highway. Once the city was behind us, in the dusk I could see peaceful farms...surrounded by barbed wire fences.

"Dad, I'd like to talk with you about the research Dr. Jackson wants me to *volunteer* for." I emphasized the word. It was the essential ingredient of my argument.

"What about it?"

"I'm not volunteering." We drove several miles in silence.

"Your mom and I will talk about it." Dad's voice was flat and resolute.

"Dad, why would you and Mom talk about something that doesn't concern you? This is about me." Inside my stomach the swallows were returning to Capistrano.

Dad sighed. More silence.

"Rachel, anything that concerns you, concerns us." This came self-righteously from Mom's side of the car.

"No, Mom, it doesn't. You are not going to be in the hospital for a week, you are not going to have IV needles stabbed in your arms, and you are not going to be made sick by an experimental drug. You aren't going to give up a full week of your summer vacation to be a prisoner!" Tears stung my eyes as I yelled.

"When *we* do this, either your father or I will give up a week of our summer vacation to be in Columbia while you're in the hospital. This research could help millions of people with diabetes. You need to think about that." Mom's voice had switched to her "I'm-a-good-parent-and-you-are-a-foolish-child" tone. Her logic was the same as for cleaning my dinner plate; it could magically save starving children in third world countries.

"So what you're saying is you don't care what's good for me." The edge on my voice was a butcher's knife, and I used it to cut a slice of her out of my life.

"Oh, Rachel, you're just a child. You're too little to understand what this really means."

I wanted to snort audibly and tell her she was too *stupid* to see what it means. I seethed with hatred for her deaf ears, and the rest of her, too.

Summer wore on. In the pit of my stomach, I knew I would not win this fight. Being a thinker, however, I had to keep coming up with possible solutions. I considered running away from home; the problem was where to run. If I went to my grandparents', they would deliver me back to my parents. If I went to stay with a friend, sooner or later, her parents would get wise and return me home, as well. Could I make it on my own living out in a field with cattle, and sneaking into farmhouses at night to plunder food? Maybe Tommy could help me. He loved to hunt animals and have them for dinner. But then, his mom usually cooked them for him, and she would turn me in for sure. Living in the wild would be especially hard, since I had to test my urine four times a day and take shots and regulate how much and what kind of food I ate.

I thought long and hard. Maybe I could hide in the church basement. I would hide in a closet, and eat leftovers from carry-in dinners. In the end it was always the same; somehow I'd be returned to my parents.

The final night came. Tomorrow I would be delivered to the Research Wardens. Mom and Dad were in the living room. Dad's face was in the newspaper and Mom read a book.

I walked in quietly and faced them both. "I'm not going tomorrow."

Dad lowered his paper; he seemed to be listening.

Mom lowered her book. "Don't be silly, of course you are. It won't be as bad as you're making it. In the afternoons you'll have free time and it will be fun. Dr. Jackson said you'll get to do crafts and go for walks. That doesn't sound so bad, now does it?" Plastic Mommy was back, in all her condescending glory.

"I'm not being silly. I'm not going. I do not volunteer, and I'm not going."

"Rachel, we've been through this before. You *are* going, and I'm done talking about it. *Go get packed!*" Her eyes flashed fire.

Dad remained strangely silent. Why didn't he protect me? Many things I had believed dissolved into nothingness.

I rounded to Mother's glare. "Then you are hideous, and I hate you more than I can ever say. The minute I can escape from your jail, I will." The words were quiet, ice cold, and unflinching. I turned and silently walked upstairs to my room.

I packed. My stomach churned. Tears fell on the clothes in my suitcase. I meant every word, and I would find a way out as soon as possible. This was not a safe place for me.

My alarm need not have rung. I had lain like a board all night. I got up and dressed in silence. Janis had gone to stay with Granny, so I had our room to myself. I heard Mom and Dad in the next room, and then someone knocked on my door.

I did not answer.

The knock came again.

If only I could become invisible and be gone when the door opened! Or if I could get out the window and run away.

The door opened. "Rachel?" It was Dad.

I stared at him wordlessly. Might he have come to rescue me?

"Are you ready to go?"

No rescue.

Dad sighed. "We'll be ready to go in a half hour."

I continued to stare at him. "Then get my bag." I pointed at my suitcase: closed, locked, and standing by the window...probably looking for a way out, too.

I walked past him and down the stairs. I weighed and measured my breakfast and ate before they came down. I would not share a meal with these people. I strode quietly out to the front porch and sat on the steps. A few cars went by; the world was waking up. This was the world of free people, people who could come and go as they pleased, people who did not exist under someone else's power, people who could choose their lives. I put my face in my hands and wept.

The three-hour trip to the research facility (which is forever embedded in my mind as the "Researchorium"…similar to the Crematorium in Auschwitz) in Columbia, Missouri, was very quiet. Mom and Dad chatted about their plans to stay in Columbia for a few days for "R and R", whatever that was. Rather obviously neither "R" stood for Research. Janis and Holly were staying with Granny, so they were probably happily watching I Love Lucy as I wheeled toward solitary confinement. I did not speak unless spoken to, and then in monosyllabic responses. My love for words would not be wasted on these people.

We arrived at the Researchorium around noon. Good timing: I could go in, dismiss my parents and eat without them. Eating was a social event in our family, and these people no longer were my family.

We checked in at the front desk. After mounds of paperwork I reached for my suitcase. Dad reached for it at the same time, and our eyes met. His gaze was soft and sad. I met it with cold steel, and yanked the suitcase toward me. "Pick me up in a week." I white knuckled my suitcase and walked after the nurse. Hopefully my actions gouged them. The pit of my stomach held a massive glacier.

My room had two single hospital beds and looked like something from a Ben Casey show. All that hit my eyes and nose reeked of sterility. The floors were so slick you could do surgery on them. For all I knew, maybe they did. I unpacked and looked out the window. Mom and Dad's car was gone. I did not want them here, but I did not want them to vanish either. I pushed my face against the warm glass and closed my eyes. Maybe I could find a world behind my eyes that was friendlier than the one in front.

Diabetes had brought new hardness into my life: hardness in terms of difficulty, as well as hardness that replaced any softness. In terms of responsibility I was an adult, but certainly not in terms of freedom. I wiped tears on my sleeve and came face-to-face with my hospital bracelet. It made me think of dog tags worn by soldiers. What was this war I fought? Who was the enemy: my parents? Diabetes? Doctors? All of the above? How could I win against an unknown It?

Dinner came. Night came. Sleeping in a hospital is like trying to rest in a haunted house; the noises are startling, but not half as terrifying as the silence. Finally, dawn pushed gray streaks across the sky, and I realized the phantoms I feared would soon materialize. I got up and dressed in my red and brown plaid dress, the one that made me look slimmer and older.

The door opened and a tall skinny nurse pushed in a rattling cart filled with tubes, bags, syringes and needles, as she dragged IV poles behind her. "Hello! Are you all ready for your big day?" She wore the indelible Witch hat nurse cap.

I thought I might faint. I sat on my bed and watched her, hoping she felt the poison darts I rammed into the invisible voodoo doll, made in her likeness.

The door opened again, and this time a tall skinny man came in. He looked like a scarecrow in a lab coat. He had a large red blotch on his face, probably the Mark of the Beast. He also had a huge grin with an expression that looked like he was headed to a party.

"So! Are you all ready?" He looked down at me from a height that had to be over six feet.

"I have no choice in this, so it doesn't matter if I'm ready, does it?"

"You know, I have diabetes, too! So we're both in this together." He continued grinning. He was like a dog trying to get approval: wagging his tail too hard, jumping on people, tottering over small children. "Well, I'll let the nurse fix you up, and I'll check back later!" He dashed out the door.

So much for "...being in this together."

"Lay down with your head at the foot of the bed, and your feet on the pillow. The drug may make you dizzy and having your feet up will help." This directive came from Witch-hat.

I lay down, and she put a tourniquet on my left arm. It was extremely tight, and pinched. My hand turned blue; my fingers went numb.

She thumped my forearm repeatedly, mumbling something about "…trying to get the veins to stand up."

Stand up? Anyone trying to stand in this room would be trodden.

She wiped my arm with an icy alcohol swab. "You'll feel a little bee sting."

I knew that was the precursor to the needle being rammed into my arm.

She stabbed.

I felt the familiar slicing, then probing, and a warm trickle of blood running down each side of my arm. I prayed she hit pay dirt.

"Well, it looks like that vein blew. We'll have to try again."

I squeezed my eyes shut. In the world behind my eyes there was a battlefield. In front of me stood two parallel rows of robots that looked like familiar people: my parents, Scarecrow doctor, Witch-hat. To win the war I had to get my life back. The only way to do that was to overcome the robots. I walked between the rows and spit on them. It was comforting. Life in my head was becoming a familiar exit for me.

"…you'll feel a little bee sting…". She stabbed me again, this time in the right arm. The pain shot from my elbow to my shoulder, and I jerked involuntarily.

"DON'T MOVE!" She had the gall to yell.

I raised my head. "You are HURTING ME!"

She met my eyes, seemingly surprised to see a human being looking at her from the other side of her needle.

"Oh…I'm sorry…sorry. I think we've got it this time." She hooked up the IV tubing and taped the needle to my arm. Then she taped my arm to a padded board.

"Why are you doing that?"

This time I got no eye contact, she looked only at the IV bag. "So you won't move your arm and disturb the needle. We'll take it off when we're done."

Webster's dictionary defines rape as, "an act or instance of robbing or despoiling or carrying away a person by force; an outrageous violation". I was being gang-raped by the Medical Machine.

Her words hung in my brain: "...so I ...wouldn't disturb *the needle*." Disturbing the needle held precedence over disturbing me. And she said, "We'll take it off..." We? Using the plural pronoun somehow removed her participation, as when a mob sets fire to a building: all are responsible for the destruction, but individuals claim personal innocence.

Cold spread up my arm as fluid drained from the bag into me. Suddenly I felt a tidal wave of nausea. I leaned forward, "I feel sick."

Witch-hat looked my direction, but avoided my eyes. "I'll get you an emesis basin." She opened my bedside table and pulled out a green, plastic, dish shaped like a comma. She put a towel on the bed to the right of my face, and placed the dish beside my mouth. "If you have to vomit, just hold the dish to your face and vomit into it."

I wondered how I would hold the dish to my face with my arm strapped to a board and invaded with an IV needle I was not supposed to disturb. I did not want to throw up, but if I did, I knew where I'd aim.

"The nausea will pass after the first twenty minutes or so. Then you'll be fine." Witch-hat announced this with the comforting tone of The Mummy. I wondered about her comprehension of twenty minutes, as she sat comfortably in a chair sipping her coffee, versus my comprehension lying with my feet in the air, stab wounds in each arm, ready to barf.

Scarecrow bustled into the room, bumping into the IV pole on his way to my bed.

With my feet raised, my dress had slid up, so I was not only sick and miserable, but also exposed. I tugged at my dress with my wounded left hand.

"So! How are we doing?"

That "we" thing again. I was too sick to answer.

"Hm. You don't look too good, a little green." He aimed his evaluation in my general direction. "We can't give you medication for the nausea, as it will contaminate our research..." His voice trailed off as though all options for comfort were nonexistent. "Well, the nausea usually subsides within the first half hour of medication, so you'll be fine." These words were aimed absentmindedly at the air about two feet above me.

I pictured what he would look like on a meat platter, roasted, with an apple in his mouth. I also noted he said the nausea might stop after a half hour, instead of twenty minutes. Did he and Witch-hat really know how long it would last? Stupid question; they had never experienced it.

I thought back to Jenny and my conversation from my first hospitalization. *"What if they don't really know what to do for diabetes? What if they're wrong?"* Oh Jenny, if you could only see me now.

Lessons Learned:

1. Research is touted as a volunteer activity. Do not believe the touters.
2. Parents you have known for many years can change in the blink of an eye, when under the influence of Strong Medicine.
3. Medical people use words in a special way that fools them into believing they do not inflict pain on their prey.

CHAPTER 13

"How much longer will this last?" I addressed Witch-hat.

"Will what last?"

"Today's research."

"About two more hours. Why?"

Why?! That deserved no answer. Two more hours of this, times four more days. I supposed it was easier than being crippled. It was even easier than having cancer. Both of those had to do with being handed a life sentence of unspeakable awfulness, so in comparison, this was not so bad. I felt no better.

My thoughts were interrupted by a jolt of nausea. I turned toward the basin, knocked it over, and threw up in the direction of Witch-hat. Green, empty-stomach-vomit poured her direction. Before she could move I made a second deposit of frothy vile liquid that landed on her arm and lap. She knocked over her coffee, which mixed with the green stuff, making a really wretched pond on her previously white skirt.

"Ahh!" She jumped to her feet. Green and brown slime ran down her skirt, over her white nylon-clad legs, and into her white shoes.

I raised my head to get the full picture. Bull's eye! My jubilation was interrupted by a sudden coldness. I shivered and sweated at the same time. It was a new misery, but did not quell my glee at having bespoiled Witch-hat. One Witch down, one Scarecrow to go.

Witch-hat cleaned up the mess, and gave me a couple of blankets. Apparently chills were a side-effect of the experimental drug they had forgotten to share with me.

"We're done for today, Rachel. Sorry it's been hard on you. Maybe tomorrow will be better." Witch-hat looked down at me from her vantage point. She ripped tape off my arm; the needle was next. I was scared to watch, but more scared not to. She held the hub and slowly pulled out the catheter, like a dagger from a sheath. Then she pressed the cotton ball into my arm with the intensity of the Dutch boy plugging a dike.

"I can hold that!" I grabbed for the cotton ball.

"Okay...well be sure to press firmly."

"Yeah, yeah. Can you just put some tape on this so I can get up?"

Witch-hat gave me eye contact. Her facial features did not contribute to emotional display. Her lips were thin, her eyes were little and set close together, and she had wrinkles on her forehead that stayed there all the time, not just when she frowned. Or maybe she frowned all the time.

She put a thick strip of tape across the cotton ball and anchored it to my arm, then tore off another strip and came at me.

"Stop! One's enough." I had sacrificed enough skin to the adhesive gods for one day.

Witch-hat stopped. "It's very important to hold pressure on the bandage for twenty minutes, and leave the tape on for at least one hour."

"Sure, no problem." I put my finger on the cotton ball to feign holding pressure. My arm was too sore to hold pressure anywhere near it, and I had succumbed to enough pressure for one day.

Witch-hat gathered her paraphernalia, loaded her metal cart, collected her IV poles and rattled out of the room. "I'll see you tomorrow."

I took that as a warning.

I was free for about twenty hours, but what did free mean in a place like this? I sat up slowly, feeling drained. As I pushed to stand, the room swayed. I leaned on the bed until it righted itself. I had to get out of this room; out of this building. A couple of exploratory steps moved me to a nearby chair - swaying, leaning, deep breathing in, let it out. My head cleared a bit. What a morning.

I walked into the hallway, and headed for the exit sign. Must get fresh air... I rear-ended the door, protecting my arms. Warm sunlight hit my face as I tottered down the steps. I was behind the Researchorium. Ahead of me were tall trees, and a grassy slope that led down to a babbling little creek. What a delight! I had just exited the Twilight Zone.

I crept down the hill and dipped my fingers in the water. It was ice cold and snapped some life into me. I sat down and took off my shoes, sticking my toes in the water. I started to feel free. Would I have felt such enjoyment if my morning had been different? Wiggling my toes in the icy water, I brushed the smooth stones underfoot. The creek was only inches deep and crystal clear. Sunshine soaked through my grown-up dress, and into the depths of my frozen heart. I closed my eyes, and let a little tear trickle down my cheek. I was so lonely. So incredibly lonely. I looked at my bruised arms, and wondered where they would jab the IV tomorrow.

The same questions I had all summer circled in my mind, but no answers surfaced. One thing was certain: I would never allow my parents the freedom to be as close to me as they had in the past. From now on, I would protect myself from them, because they were not who I thought they were. No, indeed, they were not.

I pulled my feet from the creek and rubbed them on the grass. A gentle breeze stirred the trees overhead, and I looked up. A million green leaves made a fishnet canopy, letting through diamonds of sunlight. I had believed in God since...well...forever. God was easier to feel in the sunshine than in the Researchorium. I lay back in the grass and looked at the sky. It was vivid blue, like the blue in Granny's china teacup. And it was huge. Suddenly I realized...there were no fences in the sky. As long as I could see the sky, I was *free*!

Tomorrow I would remember that when the Research Wardens came. I closed my eyes and practiced imagining the sky. There it was, blue as my Granny's teacup and going on forever...

"Rachel! There you are! We couldn't find you anywhere. Are you okay?" Mother rushed at me looking panicked, which would have been scary, had I not seen it so often before. This wasn't how I wanted to be roused.

"What do you want?"

"We were worried! No one knew where you were! You gave us such a start!"

I looked away. I had no intention of playing into her little panic game. It did not prove to me she cared, just that she *wanted* to prove she cared.

"What are you doing out here?"

"What does it matter to you what I'm doing out here?" I hoped my eyes shot fire.

"Well...your father and I wanted to take you over to the dairy where he used to work in college. He's waiting in the car and sent me to get you. His boss from college days still owns the dairy, and said we could take a tour. Then we could get chocolate malts after that!" She sounded genuinely excited, it wasn't Plastic mommy chat.

Part of me wanted to go, but that would be consorting with the enemy. "A dairy? No thanks. You seem to have forgotten that I'm diabetic. I can't have chocolate malts."

That got her. She wilted like a pansy in August.

"Oh...well...I, um...your dad and I thought you might like it. Dad will be really disappointed if you don't go." She looked at the ground.

A rusty knife blade turned inside me. She felt badly, I could tell. Well, too bad; too late for that now. But why did my stomach hurt so much?

She was right about Dad. I knew he would like to take me on a tour in the dairy. He had talked about it before. He almost took a job there when he got out of college, but he and Mom felt it would be better to raise their family in a small town, so they had moved to Memphis, Missouri, twenty-one hundred people, Saaaaahhh-LUTE! They should have stayed closer to the city. At least there were things to do, like going to the movies. There were fun places to eat, stores, and there were lots of lights. The city did not roll up the streets at five o'clock like at home. My resolve to fight grew stronger.

"I'm not interested."

What was Mother's look? Anger? Sadness? Irritation? "Rachel, we'd like to make this fun for you."

"HA! THAT's a good one!" I was yelling. "Fun is NOT what this is, and your pitiful attempts will not help. I am not interested, and I will not go." I stood up and ran a safe distance from her, bracing my back against a tree. What I wanted more than anything else was for her to run to me, throw her arms around me, say she was taking me out of this Hell-Hole, and that she would never let anyone hurt me again.

She did not.

"Rachel, you are *so unappreciative*! It will hurt your father that you're not going. Think how *I* feel about this! We're trying to do something *nice* for *you*! You are just a child and too little to understand; someday you'll know how hard it is to be a parent."

I turned away and waited for her to stop. There it was: quiet. I waited. Maybe she had gone. I turned back. Darn, still there!

"Your father and I want you to go with us to the dairy. We think you'll like it."

"You've been wrong before, and it looks like you are again." I leaned into the tree.

"All right for you." Mother's tone was icy. "I'll let your father know. He will be deeply hurt." She put her hands on her hips. She was playing the Dad-card. Dad and I got on better than she and I did, so this was her trump.

"Good idea."

She looked away, then back, "Are you sure, honey?" This time she pleaded.

I would not answer. I was exhausted with the haggling, demanding, and pleading. I cut another slice of her from my life. It eased the pain in my stomach.

Mom turned to go. "We'll have a wonderful time, and you'll be sorry you didn't come!" She squared her shoulders and marched away.

Relief flooded me, but anxiety swept in on its tails. I was obviously being a bad daughter, and Dad would be disappointed. Disappointing Dad was *not* something I wanted to do. But why did he not ask me himself? Why didn't he protect me from the Research Wardens? One bellow of his voice would clear a room, but he kept silent. He was not who I thought he was, but I had no new vision. I lay back in the grass and let the sun wash over me. Maybe it could warm my stony heart.

"Rachel?" A woman in a pastel yellow smock stood over me. A blue skirt fell in soft folds beneath the smock, and nothing on her looked sterile. Yet something told me she worked for the Researchorium. "It's three o'clock. Time for your snack."

"Three o'clock?" I sat up groggily. "Who are you?" If she was right I had not only forfeited breakfast for the research, but had also missed lunch, and slept for two hours. It was the most peaceful sleep I'd had for a long time.

"I'm Mazy, and I'm the arts and crafts director. The nurse asked me to come get you. After your snack, would you like to do a craft?" Her voice was soft, and her face looked soft, too. She smiled, even while she talked. As she spoke her blue eyes crinkled at the corners looking like rays coming off the sun. Wow. I had the urge to snuggle into her arms.

I started to get up and Mazy helped me to my feet. I stretched, still looking at Mazy. What a wonderful name. Maaaaaa-zeeee. It rolled off your tongue lighter than air.

"Are you hungry?"

"No, not really. My stomach still feels sick from this morning."

"Some of that research is hard, isn't it?"

I gave her a little smile. "It's more than hard."

Mazy put her arm around my shoulders and gave me a squeeze. "Let's forget about that now. What artsy-craftsy stuff would you like to do?"

And that is when I met Mazy. She was a retired art teacher who loved being around kids. She told me she learned more from the kids she taught, than she ever learned in art school. She said kids were the new brilliance coming into the world that would build onto the brilliance of those who came before. Mazy believed in kids. She believed in kindness. I felt her belief in me, and though it was puzzling, it was irresistible.

After my snack Mazy taught me how to do "shrink art". That was really cool. I could trace or draw a picture on plastic stuff, cut it out, then put it into the microwave and it shrunk down to the size of a bracelet charm! She even had chains to put it on, so I made myself a charm bracelet of Peanuts characters: Snoopy, Charlie Brown, Lucy, Linus, even Woodstock.

She said tomorrow we could do pottery. I had never done pottery before. She said we would put on smocks to keep our clothes from getting messy; we would throw pottery onto the wheel and later bake it. Tomorrow while the Research Wardens tortured me, I would close my eyes and see the freedom of the blue sky (as blue as my Granny's china teacup), and imagine throwing pottery.

"Time for your urine test and shot." A young nurse had quietly come to the doorway of Mazy's craft room, and made the announcement as if declaring the winner of the Kentucky Derby. She looked about Janis' age, and had no Witch-hat-frown-lines on her forehead.

I hated to leave Mazy. She was so soft and safe. I gave her a mopey look.

She gave me her sun ray smile. "I'll be here tomorrow, and we'll throw pottery all over the place!"

How many eternities would pass before I saw her again? "Thanks, Mazy. I'll look forward to it." Tears threatened; I cleared my throat.

She put her soft arms around me, and I felt like I had been embraced by a cloud. As I rested my face on Mazy's shoulder, tears ran down my cheeks and plopped onto her smock.

"I will, too," she whispered. "Don't be afraid. I'll think about you and send prayers."

"Thanks, I'll need it." I walked toward the nurse, carrying Mazy's sun ray smile in the world behind my eyes.

I did my urine test, recorded the results, and drew up my insulin. The young nurse seemed pleasant enough as she watched me draw up the insulin, but as we walked to my room the trouble started. According to my shot rotation chart, it was time to give the insulin in my arm. At home, Janis always helped me with that, and I would help her back. I explained this to the Young Nurse as we entered my cell (hospital room).

"No, you'll have to give your shot to yourself. I have to make sure you can do it." She sat down in the only comfortable chair in my room and watched me.

"Why is that?"

"We have to be sure you can inject yourself as part of your self-care evaluation." She smiled and continued to be of absolutely no assistance.

"Look, if I couldn't do my own self-care, would I be alive right now? No. I'd be dead from diabetic ketoacidosis. So how about if you help me this one time? Tomorrow, I give my shot in my leg, and that's no problem to do on my own." Her pious attitude was getting to me. I wondered if she had ever given herself a shot, especially in the arm. I doubted it.

She smiled condescendingly, and continued sitting in my comfortable chair gazing placidly at me.

I stared back. It was a High Noon stand-off.

Young Nurse began to fidget in my comfortable chair, and cleared her throat. Her condescension was not working.

I laid my insulin-filled syringe on the nightstand, crawled on my bed, and sat cross-legged, without blinking once.

Young Nurse looked toward the window. After a few moments, she looked back at me. "You have to give your insulin, you know. You can't eat dinner until you've had your shot and waited a half hour for the insulin to take effect."

I had explained my situation and requested help; there was no more to say. Then I had an idea. "Tell you what. I'll give you a shot in the arm to prove I know how, then you give me my shot." I hopped off the bed, grabbed my syringe and moved toward her.

Young Nurse sprang from the chair at lightning speed. "No, *NO!* That's not how we do things." She held her hands in front of her, and backed toward the wall...fast.

"Really?" I stepped closer.

"No, you need to give your *own* shot! Okay, how about I give your shot in your arm tonight, and tomorrow night you can give your shot in your leg?"

"Good idea." I handed her the syringe and alcohol wipe. "If you need help, I can walk you through this."

She was too shaken to appreciate the sarcasm.

Her hands were icy as she touched my arm. Good! May she never again try to use her condescension and superior attitude on me or any other patient. May she remember we are human beings, and but by the grace of God, she could be in our shoes. May she have nightmares tonight about me overpowering her and stabbing *her* arm with a syringe.

She finished my shot and turned toward the door. "Your dinner will be here in a half hour."

"I'll be here." What I wanted to say was, *Don't let the door hit your butt on the way out.* I reclaimed my comfortable chair. May God have mercy on these idiots, for they know not what they do.

Lessons Learned:
1. Nature heals just by being there.
2. Maa-zee is a lovely name.
3. Young Nurse(s) and Scarecrow doctors, like unripe fruit, should be put in storage until they have fully matured.

CHAPTER 14

Morning Two went much like Morning One with three marvelous exceptions.

1. Witch-hat got my IV started with only one stick. It hurt, but it was only one.
2. The experimental drug made me only half as sick as on Morning One. I did not get as dizzy, and I did not puke.
3. They could not scare me anymore. I had seen their worst, and I could handle it.

I remembered seeing a T-shirt one time on a guy who looked like a Hell's Angels-type that said: *Yea, though I walk through the valley of the shadow of death, I will fear no evil.* I was puzzled about a scripture verse on a shirt worn by such a rough-looking character, until I saw the back: *...for I am the meanest son-of-a-bitch in the valley.* It was my new motto.

Idiot Scarecrow doctor came in and pranced around a bit, but he was less cocky and less repulsive. He announced that tomorrow, Morning Three, was the "wash out" day for the "crossover study".

"What does that mean?"

"The first two mornings we give you one drug, the third day you can't have any drugs at all, as it will contaminate the second part of the research we'll do on Thursday and Friday, when we give you a different drug."

"Oh." I caught two impressions: one, that Wednesday they couldn't torture me – but – two, it wasn't for my recuperation, it was so I would not *contaminate* their study. To hell with their research. I had heard Dad say things like that before in a really loud voice.

The light filtering through the end of the tunnel was this: Wednesday I was scott-free and Friday afternoon I would go home, where I would continue planning my escape. That left only Thursday and Friday mornings for torture. Things were looking up.

After lunch I walked to the crafts room to throw pottery. As I threw it I would pretend it was Idiot Scarecrow, Witch-hat or Young Nurse. All of them deserved to be thrown.

"It's so good to see you!" Mazy hurried over, giving me a soft hug. She wore her pastel yellow smock, smiling her sun ray smile. If humans could view an angel, it would look like Mazy.

Her hug melted my Hell's Angels attitude, and pent up tears oozed out.

"You're crying. Are you okay?"

I tried to sniff back the tears. "It's hard here. But today was better than yesterday, and I have tomorrow off, so that's good, right?"

"Right." Her eyes were soft.

"Mazy, let's throw pottery."

"You got it." She patted my cheek and started pulling out all kinds of strange and interesting pieces of equipment.

I learned that you do not actually throw pottery, as one would throw plates to break them. You kind of toss it onto the potter's wheel and make bowls and plates, pitchers and other stuff. It was wonderfully messy and fun. Making a mess in this ridiculously sterile place was sheer poetry, and doing it with Mazy was magic. She seemed to enjoy making a mess even more than I did.

By the time we were done, her pastel yellow smock was soggy and gray-brown. We put all the pieces we made into a really hot oven called a kiln. They would roast overnight and be done in the morning. Kiln is a funny word, like kilt or kin, but not even close to meaning the same thing. It sounds like ilk, too, meaning sort or kind. Sometimes words make sense, sometimes they leave huge gaps asking to be filled with understanding. I could not fill the gap, so I filled the kiln.

"We did great work today, look at this! You made two bowls and three vases. That's amazing!"

"Thanks. It was really fun. Can we do it again tomorrow? I have the whole day off; I could make place settings for twelve!"

"Let's get cleaned up. Tomorrow we'll go on a long walk, have a picnic lunch, throw stones in the creek, and whatever else we want to do. How does that sound?"

"Great!"

"Wear comfy clothes and shoes, because we'll have an adventure."

We hugged. I didn't cry this time; it was progress.

The next morning dawned brilliantly. How could it not? I showered and dressed in a rush. Mazy would be here at nine o'clock, which was still two hours away, but I could not slow down. I tested my urine and went to the medication room. A new nurse was there.

"My urine test was negative and I'm ready to draw up my insulin."

The nurse looked up from the medication book. "I need to see your test to be sure it's negative. Go get it." Her voice was matter-of-fact, not mean, but not friendly.

"Too late. I already dumped it out and washed the test tube. It's upside-down, drying in the bathroom."

"How do I know it was really negative?" She became Query Nurse.

I decided she was not mean, but she thought I did not know what I was doing. (Heavy sigh.) "Because I just told you. I've been doing this for a while. I know negative when I see it." I walked to the refrigerator and pulled out my insulin bottles. "How much insulin is ordered for this morning?"

"Eight NPH and four Regular. My name is Carrie."

That was better. Now she was not Query Nurse, she was Carrie. "I'm Rachel Gifford, but I guess you know that if you know how much insulin I'm supposed to take."

Carrie watched me as I drew up the insulin. It was a complex task. First I wiped off both insulin vials with the alcohol swab, then I put eight units of air into the NPH bottle, withdrew the needle and put four units of air into the Regular. Leaving the needle in the vial, I turned it upside down and drew out four units. Next I put the needle in the NPH, making sure none of the Regular went into the NPH vial, and drew out eight units, giving me a total of twelve units of insulin. I checked my rotation chart and thankfully, it was not time for my arm. I wiped my leg with alcohol, and dried it with a cotton ball. Stabbing the needle into my leg as fast as I could, I pulled back the plunger to check for blood in case I had accidentally hit a vein. Injections should just go into my fat layer, which thankfully now was smaller than it used to be. No blood, I pushed the plunger, injecting the insulin. Removing the needle, I covered the injection site with a dry cotton ball and handed Carrie the used syringe. No more shots until dinner.

"Good job, you really know what you're doing." Carrie smiled.

"Thanks." I headed back to my room. It was nice to have someone smile at me in the medication room, the very Sepulcher of Sterility in the Researchorium. I looked at my watch. In thirty minutes I would get breakfast, and about forty minutes after that Mazy and I would start our adventure. My heart sang a little tune. It was a Sunday School song, and the last phrase was, "...now I am happy all the day!" It nearly burst from my chest.

"Are you ready for an adventure?" It was Mazy! Breakfast was done and I had asked the nurse to pack my morning and afternoon snack, along with my lunch, so Mazy and I could take it with us. I also packed my urine tester. With the food and tester we would not need to come back until dinner. Yahoo!

"I am very ready! C'mon, we're history." And we were.

We went to a small amusement park and rode every ride we wanted to, and none that we didn't. After the amusement park we walked along a path that went through some trees, and then a glorious park with lots of shade, grass, and a wading pond. Taking off my shoes, I waded for a long time, overruling the dictum that *diabetics* are not supposed to go bare-foot.

I ate my morning snack early because I felt a reaction coming on. I was thrilled. It meant I was moving, running and being human, instead of lying on a bed being Resident Guinea Pig. I ate lunch early for the same reason. We ate in the park at a picnic table. A huge tree shaded us so we were cool as cucumbers, yet it let shimmers of light dapple across us. I was ecstatic, and at peace, all at the same time. Lunch did not get rid of the shaky low-blood-sugar-feeling, so I ate my afternoon snack, too.

"Mazy, we're going to have to get another snack for me. I'm running around so much, I've eaten all my food." I held my snack bag upside-down and shook it at her.

She laughed. "What do you want?"

An idea formed in my head. "When I'm really active at home, Mom lets me have ice cream. What do you think?"

"How much ice cream?" Mazy looked curious, not dubious.

"One or two scoops, depending on how much activity I've had." I wondered if she would doubt me, and turn into Query Mazy.

"Two it is, then! We've been running all over the place. And we'll get another snack to take with you in case you get low in the meantime."

Mazy was beyond beautiful.

We went to Baskin Robbins, and I had one scoop of butter-brickle, and one chocolate fudge. Mazy had scoops of chocolate fudge and chocolate chip. We snarfed it down like there was no tomorrow.

Tramping through yet another park, we picked up rocks, and splashed through a creek with our shoes on, getting slogging wet. We threw rocks into the water, and Mazy even taught me how to skim a stone over the surface. It was magic. It was beauty. It was joy. Until today, childhood had been many lifetimes ago.

"Mazy."

"Yeah?"

"I leave Friday. Tomorrow will be our last afternoon together." A cloud slid across the sun.

Mazy looked at me, as we sat by the rippling water on a fallen log. "Yes...in a way."

"What do you mean, 'in a way'? It *will* be. It *WILL* be the last time we're together. Tomorrow is it! They research me Friday morning and then I go home. I won't see you anymore. You may not know this, but I think you might have saved my life this week."

Mazy scooted over and put her arms around me. We sat for a while in silence. "I'll be with you always, Rachel."

"Whaddya mean?"

"Do you know the verse in the Bible where Jesus says, 'Lo, I will be with you always, even to the end of the earth?'"

I thought for a minute. I had memorized that verse for Girl's Auxiliary at church. It was part of what they called The Great Commission. Jesus was going back to heaven and his disciples were broken-hearted, but He told them not to be sad, because He would be with them always. "Yeah. Why?"

"Well, it's the same for people you love, too. No matter where you are or where they are, their spirit will always be with you. Just close your eyes and take a deep breath, and you'll know I'm right there."

Mazy's gaze floated into my heart, and warmed me. I looked down wondering if it glowed through my chest. No glowing on the outside, but inside it spread. Tears trickled down my cheeks. "You will. I know you will."

I closed the car door and walked toward the Researchorium. The Day of Adventure was over, yet it lived inside me.

"I'll see you tomorrow!" Mazy waved.

I waved back. Still warm inside, I walked into the Researchorium. When I reached my room I looked around, comparing it with the day I arrived. It was not as big or cold; the shiny tile floors looked just as slick and sterile, but softer. I sat cross-legged on my bed and thought about Mazy. I wondered if she had been afraid a lot in the past. She must have been. How else could she so expertly help me? Maybe she was an angel. What were angels? How did they get to people who needed them? Where were they the rest of the time? So many questions...they melted into my brain like ice cream.

Ice cream! What had our trip to Baskin Robbins done to my blood sugar? What if I had not exercised enough? I jumped off the bed and ran to the bathroom. I peed, tested, waited...it was blue. I cleaned my tester, and headed to the medication room. After tonight's shot I had only three more shots before I left the Researchorium. Hurrah! Yet, once I got home, I had to figure out a way to escape. Heavy sigh. I thought back to Mazy again; it was easier.

Morning Four. Same Witch-hat, same Idiot Scarecrow Doctor...same 'ol, same 'ol. On some counts my luck held, on others it failed. They stabbed me three times before getting the IV in. I wondered at their incompetence. Idiot Scarecrow Doctor came in less than before; I counted it a blessing. The experimental drug did not make me sick at all. Then I was done.

I trotted into the crafts room. "Hi Mazy."

"Hey there. Are you rested up from our Day of Adventure?"

"Yeah, no problem. It was wonderful, and you're wonderful. I'm really gonna miss you." I had not meant to just blurt it out, but there it was... hopped out like a toad.

"Me, too. You're one in a million." She gave me a soft hug.

"Hey, you know what? My urine test was negative when we got back, so we did exactly the right thing with the ice cream. Cool, huh?"

"Of course we did. You know what to do for your diabetes."

Her faith in me was so...uncommon. I was suddenly energized. "Let's be artsy-craftsy. What should we do today?"

"I have an idea. How about if we make clay people and animals and then tell each other a made up story about them?"

"That's a funny idea. Let's do it."

We made donkeys, cows, sheep, cats, dogs, houses, trees, kids, and even a few grown ups. But not many. In my estimation, the fewer grown ups, the better. We made up funny stories, ridiculous stories, long stories and short stories. We flew our clay characters around on brooms, magic carpets and clouds. They went magical places that we made up ourselves. We made it all up. We even made up clothes for our characters and described the colors, the trim, the flow of the garment, even the fabric. Some were made of leaves and tree twigs, others of butterfly wings or "fairy fiber" that glistened in the sun like a diamond.

Then it was over.

"Mazy?"

"Yes."

"I'm really sad."

We sat at a low table surrounded by our newly created clay characters who had just lived their first afternoon of life. She scooted close and put her arm around my shoulder.

"When you said you'd always be with me I felt warm inside. I still do. Is that coming from you, or is it just me?"

Mazy snuggled closer. "Both, baby...both. I gave you a spark of love, and it lit yours."

No one had called me baby for a long time. In fact, I usually considered it a criticism, but not the way Mazy said it. Her "baby" sounded beautiful and soft, like a baby kitten.

Friday morning came: Day Five. Witch-hat came, but Idiot Scarecrow did a no-show. That was a gift. One stab got the IV in, and the experimental medication only made me a little dizzy. It was over.

Such mixed feelings: glad to leave prison, but scared to go home. My relationship with Mom and Dad had changed forever. Then there was Mazy. A sharp jab went through my chest, but she was right about the spark. Whenever I thought of her the warm feeling came back. She would be with me always.

Lessons Learned:
1. When you're little, though most adults demand you act like a grown up, they never tire of questioning your adult behavior.
2. You can't always get what you want. But if you try sometimes, you might find...you get what you need.

A Word to the Wise: I need to tell you something about Mazy. In physical form she never existed. In fact as she appeared on my written pages I chuckled at what I was writing, and tried to stop her story. But she would not stop, she flew from my fingers, and spread across page after page. I felt like a liar as I typed, yet a bigger liar should I stop. To the best of my recollection there was an arts and crafts room at the Researchorium, and we did things with construction paper, shrink art, glue, paints, pottery and crayons. I also think we went on a field trip, but that is all I remember.

Here's what I wonder. I was in desperate need of softness, beauty, love and touch. I needed a warm, loving woman who could hear me. Did I psychologically manufacture Mazy? Was she an angel? Did the God I knew bring me the compassion I needed in dreams? In my subconscious? In my imagination? I have more questions than answers.

What I do know is that leaving Mazy out of this story would omit a truth. And it would break my heart.

PART TWO:

THE END OF THE BEGINNING

Chapter 15

Between my sixth and seventh grade years, Mom and Dad made a big decision. They both took teaching positions in Moravia, Iowa, Mom teaching grade school and Dad teaching both junior and senior high Biology, Chemistry and Physics. Moravia was more than an hour drive from Memphis, our home in Missouri, so during the week we lived in Moravia and attended school, then drove home for the weekends.

Changing schools and towns was a relief for me. Losing my long-time best friend in sixth grade had left me feeling lost, and diligently searching for a new best friend. Despite my efforts, no one applied for the job. In retrospect, I am sure I tried too hard. Rejection became a chronic low-grade fever for a while. After physically rejecting my own pancreas, I had no time to feel emotional rejection anymore...way too busy. I looked forward to a new school; a chance to start over.

This arrangement also gave my family a different lifestyle. My parents' attention scattered by living in two places, teaching during the week, and keeping up the farm on weekends. It gave me room to breathe. Besides, I still couldn't figure out a place to go where I wouldn't either die – or – be returned to my parents. I would have to bide my time.

Dad became my science teacher. That had both good and not-so-good sides to it. One not-so-good part was that Dad thought everyone in my class would believe he gave me extra privileges, so he was harder on me to disprove that theory. I had always gotten top grades, but now the pressure was on to excel not only in Biology (Dad's expectation), but all other subjects as well, so it did not appear to my classmates that I got sneak previews of the test. I walked a knife edge that sometimes cut through my shoes.

Another difficulty was Dad himself. Dad's premise on teaching was: The first semester you are the meanest Simon LaGree in the school system. After the kids learn to respect (fear) you, you can let up. Heavy sigh. With some kids I became evil by association.

Those not-so-good items were further complicated by the fact that Dad was brilliant. Brilliant people are not always the best teachers. If their pupils are brilliant, it works great. It the pupils are struggling, a brilliant person may not be able to come down to their level. Complicate that with the mere fact that we were seventh graders, and you get the picture. Suffice it to say, my first several months at Moravia were tenuous.

So what was the good part of this? I could keep an eye on Dad. Dad had his first heart attack when I was seven years old. His second was when I was eleven. Each time the doctors told us if he made it through the first night we would be lucky, and thereafter it was a day at a time. Over the years, I appointed myself Dad's guardian angel. It was my job to keep him alive.

Why would a small child think such a thing? Who the heck knows? Part of it was self-preservation. Mom and I had difficulties getting along, and Dad was my link to the family. If something happened to him, my future was uncertain. Not only that, in today's terms Dad could be called a rage-aholic. He was never physically violent, but his outbursts were big, loud, terrifying and frequent. The doctors had warned that if he got angry it could bring on another heart attack (kill him). When Dad raged, I could talk him down. I would go to him and sit quietly for a while. Then I would start chit-chat of some sort, constantly monitoring his reactions, and pretty soon he was calm again.

Over time this job moved from self-appointment to a family opportunity. When Mom or my siblings wanted something from Dad, I would be summoned to make the request, as I was more likely to get a "yes" answer.

This being the case, having class for one hour every day with Dad gave me the opportunity to be sure he was doing okay. If I sensed he needed help, I was there. For some reason, as a child, this did not seem heavy; it seemed right, and gave me a place to belong in the family. You might think all this added stuff would make me hate the school change. You would be wrong. Anything new brought promise for me. New people, new classes, new things to learn – I needed fresh air.

Moravia had a junior high girl's basketball team. I had no prior experience with basketball, but the idea intrigued me. However, basketball practice held some conundrums. Practice took place after school around the time my morning NPH peaked, which meant extra exercise would make my blood sugar drop like a rock. Mom and I were not sure how much food I would need for the extra exercise of practice, so the first day we packed two sandwiches, a banana and a thermos of milk. Mom said if that was not enough, I should tell the coach to stop practice, because he was working us too hard. Right. Mom was pretty funny sometimes.

My stomach fluttered with butterflies the entire school day before our evening practice. I thought of Tommy. He had played basketball in highschool. I wondered if he got butterflies, too. Probably not.

When the last bell rang I ran four blocks to the gymnasium, streaked into the locker room, and started changing as fast as I could. To save time, I ate while I changed. I bit off a huge chunk of sandwich. The bread was sandpaper, and the roast beef was pure sinew. No matter how hard I chewed the wad in my mouth grew. Girls in the locker room looked at me funny. Finally I spit the awful goo into the toilet and started again. Half the sandwich was gone by the time I tied my high tops. The banana was next and slid down more cooperatively. Drinking a thermos of milk seemed like the sure road to barfing, so I vetoed that. I grabbed the other half sandwich and headed for the drinking fountain, hoping water would help. It did. I shoved the sandwich remains into my mouth, slurped water like a dehydrated camel, and came up for air.

That is when Mrs. Smith came for a drink.

Mrs. Smith taught music, and also was the mom of an eighth-grade girl on the basketball team. Her eyes widened as she watched my mouth grind furiously, cheeks puffed out like a chipmunk, water dripping off my chin.

"My, you must *really* be hungry!" She looked shocked.

I tried to speak, but my tongue was immobilized. She continued to stare as I slurped more water and finally downed a huge chunk.

"I'm diabetic. I have to finish this sandwich before basketball practice. Coach says if we're late to practice, don't bother coming." I slurped more water and finally the glob dropped into my stomach like a target missile. I straightened, nodded at Mrs. Smith, and took off down the hall. No doubt she thought I was an impolite freak of nature, and though I hated that, it was secondary to getting to practice.

Practice was three hours of non-stop exercise. It was fun, but nerve-racking. I could not tell if my jitters were from low blood sugar, exhaustion or just being in continuous "freak-out" mode. I decided to keep moving, and if the jitters were low blood sugar, pretty soon I'd lose energy. Then I would eat. I did not want to stop practicing to eat, as I was sure it would not bode well for making the team. I was not the worst player there, but certainly not the best.

When practice finally ended I took inventory of our team wannabes. We all looked like we had been through a wringer. Maybe I was no more tired or apprehensive than the others...? Having diabetes always made me feel as if I stuck out like a sore thumb. I put amazing energy into trying to look like "all the others", as though being nondiabetic gave a normality that allowed "them" to all look the same. Dr. Jackson was right. I could do anything anybody else could do, I just had to plan more, think more and work harder than everybody else. So far, so good.

After several weeks of practice, I started to have a better feel for how much to eat, and ate as I walked the four blocks to the gym. Everything is easier when you know what to expect. Amazingly enough, I made the team. I even made "A" level, which meant I got to wear the cool starter uniform. Though I started very few games, I did play in a few others after we racked up a big score.

Initially, games were another nightmare. First of all, I never knew if, or how long, I might play, so I had no idea how much to eat beforehand. In the beginning I usually ate too much and my urine test was four plus afterward. Very irritating. As I got better at guessing how much to eat, I also got better at basketball. Then I played more, and did not eat enough. This is the tight wire called diabetes.

At least I never had to call a time out to eat. That might have been more humiliation than I could have endured. Each game had a limited number of time-outs, and if I called a time-out that threw off Coach's plan, we might lose. I could envision my popularity in such a case.

Junior high saw the beginning of orthodontics. Like I needed one more thing. That was a funny thing about life: it didn't ask what I wanted. Or maybe I was deaf...or it was. I thought it would have been a nice option to job-share diabetes. For example, maybe Mom or Dad could take diabetes for a few days and give me a break. Nice idea, but no prize.

Well, back to braces...at least they did not require I go to the hospital. Everything was done by office visits. The beginning was scary, because I had to have teeth pulled. I was fairly certain that would not be an enjoyable experience. I also wondered how I could stay on my meal plan after my teeth were pulled.

It took juggling of exchanges, with scrambled eggs becoming my main meat exchange for a while. After the teeth were pulled, the rest was downhill, except for the time I tried to catch a basketball with my face. That required existing for a few days on soup swilled through a straw, but compared to the vigilance required by diabetes, braces were small potatoes.

Living in a small town meant going to a specialist physician incurred a road trip. Depending on the variety of doctor, the trip could be thirty minutes to three hours one way. Mom liked to spice up trips with shopping events. There was a huge Wholesale Grocery Market in Ottumwa, Iowa, where Mom took me to the orthodontist. She often paired the Wholesale Market as our shopping event.

At one appointment we had an exceptionally long wait. Mom decided to save time by going to the Market while I waited to see the orthodontist. Off she went, and I waited. One thing about Mom's shopping trips; when she shopped she forgot about time. My appointment started, proceeded and ended, but Mom was nowhere in sight. It was near lunchtime, and never being one to cool my heels, I devised a plan. I would walk toward the Market, flag down Mom as she drove back to the office, and we'd go have lunch. It was a beautiful spring day, and a walk would be great.

I breezed out of the building and toward the four-lane road Mom would take to come get me. I breathed in the smell of lilacs and it put a cloud under me. I was out of school, my appointment was over for another month; I was a free girl. I flitted along on the median between the four lanes of traffic watching for Mom's blue car.

After twenty minutes of walking, I was hot and getting hungry. About that time I realized my purse, carrying my candy supply for low blood sugar, was in Mom's car. Worry prickled down my neck, along with sweat. I felt shaky, but wasn't sure if it was from worry or low blood sugar. Where was Mom? What if I couldn't make it all the way to the Market?

Then I saw her blue car. Relief rushed through me as I waved my hands at her. The car did not slow down. I jumped up and down and waved my hands. No response. I yelled, jumped up and down, and waved my arms, nearly falling off the median. Mom sped past me. Dread fell into my stomach and flopped around. Surely she would come back? I turned and stared after the blue car as it disappeared over the hill.

This was very much not a good thing. I walked back toward the orthodontist office. I could tell my blood sugar was dropping. I stumbled and my tongue had gone completely numb; I had to do something fast. I looked across two blurry lanes of traffic and saw houses. They were cute little white houses with flowers around them. Surely someone nice lived in houses like that.

God, I need help. Please take me to a house where someone will help me. Tears mingled with the sweat on my face. I hated going to someone's door and asking for food. What if no one was home? What if they thought I was a beggar and called the police? What if they would not give me food? What if I passed out and went into a seizure like Janis had done so many nights? There would be no one to help me. They would not even know how to help, and I might seize long enough to have permanent brain damage. (I was well-schooled in worrying.)

The oncoming traffic slid toward me in slow motion, with whole parts of the picture missing. Low blood sugar does strange things to the brain; crossing two lanes of traffic would be tricky.

God, here I go. Please help me. I was pretty sure He heard, but it would have been nice to feel a strong hand doing the Boy Scout thing across the street. In an act of desperation I stepped off the curb. It felt like I was slogging across the deepest ocean floor. I reached forward grasping for...what? My knees buckled and I felt sharp scraping on my knees and forearms. Could I get up? I struggled forward in a half stumble-half crawl, and finally pulled myself to the curb. I could not sit long. I had to keep going...I had to find food. I stood and staggered toward the houses.

Okay, God...which house? I was exhausted and overwhelmed. I had to find a helping house fast. I lurched forward: walking, stumbling, walking, falling, walking. I reached the nearest house, and fell up the steps. As I thumped on the door, I wondered what to say when someone came. What if no one came? Could I make it to another house? The door opened, revealing a tall elderly gentleman with snow white hair.

"Hello there." He looked down at me.

I began to cry, words slurring out of my mouth. "My name iz Rashel Gifffff..erd. I have diabedes, and my blood sugar izzz really low. I need food." The words came from a deep well inside me and echoed through my head. I was not sure I spoke at all...had I only thought the words?

"My dear, come inside!" He opened the door and took my arm, pulling me inside. "Lydia, this little girl needs something to eat quickly." He pulled out a chair where I sank like the Titanic.

I could not believe my good fortune. *Thanks, God.*

Lydia was quick as a wink. She had a sandwich, milk and fresh fruit in front of me before I realized she'd left the room. I chugged the milk and gobbled the fruit, knowing they would raise my blood sugar fastest. Etiquette had left my brain, leaving only survival instincts. I imagined looking like Oliver Twist at his worst.

Slowly my vision improved, like walking out of a deep fog, and feeling tiptoed onto my tongue. Blood sugar seems to have a critical mass when rising from the ashes of hypoglycemia, at which the room almost audibly clicks into place. Suddenly I was there. I wiped at my tears, and looked clearly (fairly clearly...) at my rescuers. They were an elderly couple. They both looked worried, and Lydia kept bringing food. These people had the kind, loving look of grandparents.

"Dear, where is your mother?" Lydia subtly pushed a plate of grapes nearer my elbow.

I was befuddled. Where was she? Why wasn't she here? Then I remembered. "I don't know where she is." I told them the saga as it slipped slowly into my brain.

"So, you have diabetes?" Mr. Grandfather was looking at me compassionately.

"Yes. I've had it for a year. I'm so sorry to bother you, and I so much appreciate your help. I might have died if you hadn't helped me." A little sob escaped.

Mr. Grandfather put his arm around my shoulders and squeezed. He patted my arm. "Who is your orthodontist?"

"Dr. McDonald."

"Oh, Jim McDonald! I am a retired dentist, and I know Dr. McDonald well. His office is more than two miles from here! You walked all that way?"

I nodded.

"You poor child! No wonder you're hungry." Lydia looked aghast. The way she said "poor child" sounded like a good thing. "Lloyd here has diabetes, and he takes pills. Do you take pills?"

So, Mr. Grandfather's name was Lloyd. "No, ma'am, I take shots."

"Shots! Oh my. One in the morning?"

"No, ma'am. One a half hour before breakfast, and another a half hour before lunch."

"Oh gracious." Lydia softly patted my shoulder. "You are a very brave child."

Could I possibly have stumbled into a better house?

"Well, I'll call Jim McDonald's office and see if your mother is there. I bet she's worried." Lloyd got up and moved in grandfather gait toward the phone.

Worried? Yeah, she was probably in a veritable froth. "Yes, please. That would be wonderful. And thank you so much."

"Here, let's play checkers while Lloyd calls the office." Lydia pulled out a checkerboard and started setting up the game. "Do you want red or black?"

"Which do you prefer?"

"No, dear. You choose first."

"I'd like red, please." I hoped she didn't secretly prefer red.

"Lloyd always wants the black checkers, so this time I get them!" She gave me a wicked smile.

We were half done with the first game when Lloyd came back. "I got your mother, and she's on her way here. She was pretty worried." He glanced at the checkerboard. "Playing checkers, eh?" He chuckled. "Lydia is the Queen of Checkers. She'll skunk you."

I didn't care. I knew I was in good hands.

A couple of games later the doorbell rang. Lloyd walked to the door and ushered Mom into the living room.

"Rachel! I'm so glad to see you." Mom turned to Lloyd and Lydia. "Thank you both for your help. Thank you so much."

"Oh, it was no trouble at all. We enjoyed talking with Rachel. She's a very spunky little girl." Lloyd beamed down at me.

Lydia patted my shoulder. "She seems to know how to handle herself."

I beamed a little myself.

Mom thanked them five or six more times before getting to the door, and another two or three times as we walked to the car. I turned to take a last look at the charming white house with flowers around it. The flowers looked as soft as Lydia's hand had been on my shoulder.

As we drove toward home Mom bombarded me with questions: Why did I leave the doctor's office? Where was I? Why was I walking down the median of a busy four-lane road? What was I thinking? Then she apologized for not seeing me, as though it had been an act of negligence. I knew it wasn't.

I could not stay with her words. My mind was like black fertile loam sprouting amazing gems of wonderings. In the fog of low blood sugar, how had I stumbled across two lanes of relentless traffic without getting smashed? How had I found a house where people were home in the middle of a workday? How had I been able to keep staggering long enough to reach any house at all? How in the world had it been my good fortune to happen upon Lloyd and Lydia? And Lloyd even knew Dr. McDonald! I remembered my prayers for help. Lloyd and Lydia were more than I had needed...they were what my heart called for. Tears swam in my eyes.

Thanks, God.

Lessons Learned:

1. Every new experience threw diabetes off kilter for a while. Like basketball, with practice it got better.
2. Having braces was a pea under the mattress compared to taking care of diabetes.
3. Of all the things in the world to die from, I don't want to die from hypoglycemia.
4. There are incredibly nice people in the world, and God takes care of me. I don't know why, I just know it.

Chapter 16

In eighth grade I found out I had scoliosis. I remembered Theresa, from my hospitalization at the Medical Center, and wondered if I would soon join her flipping from front-to-back like a pancake, somewhere in the ICU. I would have panicked, had my life not already made me adrenalin-depleted.

My scoliosis was a double curve: one at the top and a counter curve at the bottom, making my spine into an "S". Now-a-days children are regularly screened in school for scoliosis, and braces are inconspicuous and can be worn discretely under clothing. Not so in the dark ages.

My first realization that something might be amiss occurred as I bent over to change into shorts in gym class.

A classmate scrutinized me and said, "Rachel, your back looks weird, have you been in a car wreck?"

I was a little shocked at her bluntness, and wanted to retort "No why? Have you?" I settled for "No," said hoity-toitly.

"You have a big hump."

Everyone in the locker room stared, and this girl quickly fell from classmate to scum-of-the-earth.

The words gnawed at me all day. That evening I told Mom what had happened.

"Well, I think your back's just fine!" She had the hoity-toity thing going, too. "Take off you sweater and let me check."

I shed the sweater. Silence. Not a good sign.

"Well, there is something here, but I'm not sure what it is. We'll just take you to the doctor and have it checked out." She acted nonchalant, which meant she was worried.

The checking-out doctor visit resulted in a later, additional trip to Columbia to the Medical Center, for yet one more specialist visit. My gut twisted, enduring more interminable waiting, x-rays, a diagnosis, and then a hideous brace (monster). The Milwaukee braces of the past had huge roll bars in the back that went from a bar under my chin to a metal encased leather girdle that rested on my pelvis like a small anchor. In between my chin and pelvis was an erector set of rods, screws and leather strappings. I named it Horace

Horace was so big, clothing had to be worn underneath unless you cared to wear a tent or awning. I did not. Mom did all she could to help, taking me shopping for wrinkle-proof tops that were soft and could be worn under Horace (wrinkle-proof stuff was not plentiful in the late 1960s unless it was tie died: not acceptable for school), and skirts big enough to fit over Horace. A sad reminder: I had just started fitting into normal size clothes. We decided I could wear a vest or sweater over the upper part of Horace. Mom made two vests and we got a couple of sweaters. Hence my wardrobe.

Problem being, Horace-the-demon-of-steel had screws on the back and soon cut through my sweaters and vests. I felt even more despicable than before. Horace (and I, by unsatisfying association) actually destroyed clothing. My clothing. My only wearable clothing.

Diabetes had allowed me to be discrete about being a Freak. Horace gave me no leeway; word was out. Trying to get into the one-piece school desks was nearly impossible. Getting out required extreme practice, and the first few times I toppled over – along with the desk. Screws on the back of Horace left scratches on wood or metal furniture and ripped upholstery; I had to be careful where I sat. Boys in my class began to yell, "Hey Roll-bars!" as I walked down the hallway. I wanted to run into the bathroom and sob to death. I was not sure I could die from sobbing, but I hoped so.

Yet I knew better than to cry. That would look like I cared, and having been fat for so long taught me above all else...*never, but never* let them know they upset you. Then the meanness never stops. Ignoring stupidity sometimes made it stop. The only problem was I could not ignore the slicing inside me.

I wore Horace twenty-three hours of every day. The doctors allowed one hour to bathe, dress and change. Generous. During this time my orthodontics intensified as well. I now had "head gear" to wear at night. Head gear consisted of a wire arc that encircled my face, hooking into slots in the bands attached to my upper molars. Attached to the arc was an elastic collar that encircled my neck and head. I never, *never* looked at myself after assembling all this each night. Who would? Had I walked into a lightening storm, I would have been fricasseed. I was more than certain if I looked up "freak" in the dictionary, there would be a picture of me. I did not look.

I was terrified Horace would knock me out of playing basketball, but grace was on my side. Doctors allowed me to remove Horace for practice, leave him in the locker room, and put him back on afterward. The same was allowed for games. I cried the first time I had to put him back on after practice. Everyone stared, or pretended not to stare as they looked away between stares. I finally retreated to a toilet cubicle, put on Horace, my clothes, and waited until everyone left. By then the room was dark. All the better: most monsters come out only after dark.

For some wonderful reason, when I had my orthopedic appointments at the medical center, I frequently got by without encountering medical students. At one fateful visit however, Dr. Litton, my orthopedic surgeon, let me know he would not be in town for my next visit, and his chief resident would see me. I was immediately overcome with apprehension. Dr. Litton was older than Dad, he was kind, and he had gray hair. God only knew what a chief resident would do with me. Surgery? Would I join Theresa?

Dr. Litton assured me the chief resident would follow "the current plan of care" without making changes.

Right.

The appointment day came, and as I sat alone in the exam room, in walked a man far too young and inexperienced to let "the current plan" ride. He looked just a little older than Tommy. He decided I needed a new gadget that would encircle my left shoulder like the yoke you see on oxen, then attach to Horace, pulling my left shoulder up and back. I was aghast.

"Dr. Litton said no changes would be made while he was away." I tried the dead-on approach.

Dr. Young & Inexperienced gave me no eye contact. "This change needs to be made. It will help train your muscles for better balance."

"Dr. Litton said no changes would be made while he was gone." Maybe he hadn't heard me.

"I'm his chief resident. If any changes need to be made, I would make them." He began to measure my arm and shoulder.

"He said no changes were to be made."

"This will only take a minute. Don't worry." He continued measuring.

I did worry. As he measured, turned me back and forth, touched parts of my body I did not want touched, I went deep inside to a place he could not reach. Sight, sound nor touch penetrated here. In this place there were no braces, and I had a voice people listened to.

"Okay, that should do it." He spoke.

I stayed in my safe place.

He shook me. "Are you okay?"

Jerking from my safety I looked at him. "It really doesn't matter, does it?"

For a moment he was caught off guard. Then he chuckled and left the room.

The shoulder yoke arrived in the mail two weeks later. Of all the things they took, I missed my voice the most.

Although Horace was a weight on me, literally and emotionally, after a while he became less problematic. He did not require anything of me after getting assembled. Kids got used to how I looked, and ridicule died down. Also, unlike diabetes, he was not *forever.* My freshman year I could take him off during school. The third year of Horace, I wore him only at night, which continued four more years. Horace went with me to college, but he really never got any smarter. Only less visible.

I wished for sage knowledge as to why I got the triple whammy of diabetes, scoliosis, and crooked teeth. Science had no answer. My parents had no answer. If God knew, He wasn't talking. There is that verse in the Bible about God not giving you more than you can bear, but I wondered if

He had checked my stamina lately. What if I bore just a little too much, and that's why I got a crumpled spine in the first place?

Thinkers love to read, especially when they have a problem. Reading about other people's lives helps distract from your own. During this time, I read a quote by Mignon McLaughlin, American author, saying, "Even cowards can endure hardship; only the brave can endure suspense." I got exceptionally brave in those years.

Slumber parties were a learning issue in junior high, often accompanied by drama. Terri was one of my friends in teen years. Her house in Memphis was two blocks from mine, only one block if you cut across the neighbor's yard. Her parents owned the busiest of three cafés in town. (Small towns do not need a lot of restaurants.) She knew about my diabetes, and it was not a big deal to her. Big relief. When we ate at her house or her parents' café she made sure we had Diet Pepsi or iced tea with Sweet 10. Sugar-free sweeteners and foods were *not* plentiful in the 1970s, so she watched out for me that way.

In contrast, at the junior high slumber parties, I was one among a crowd of giddy, giggling and often goofy young women. Mom always got nervous about slumber parties, and wanted to discuss my diabetes with the hosting Mom, which was nearly too embarrassing to endure. I could take care of myself, and had proven it many times over.

Though it was not easy. Usually, these parties had non-stop food: chips and dip, cake, cookies, ice cream, punch, pizza...you name it. It was wonderful and terrible. Also, we all know "Slumber Party" and "Sleep Over" are misnomers. No one ever sleeps. In fact, sometimes punitive action was taken upon hapless Sleeping Beauties who succumbed to exhaustion, such as dipping their hands in warm water to make them pee the bed or applying Tabasco sauce to their lips. So much for the innocence of childhood.

These days, I hear kids calling such rendezvous by more realistic names like "Stay Over" and "Overnight". Those are more depictive. Regardless, staying up all night is out of the ordinary, and for someone with diabetes it calls for a lot of improvisation. Since I now had to think like a pancreas,

I had to know what kind of insulin to take for all night activity. I also had to know when to eat more so I would not get hypoglycemic, and crash n' burn. It was an elegant juggling act that required constantly monitoring how I felt.

I synced with my body like an Olympic athlete: I could live or die by my body's cues. I had to differentiate between tired that came from non-stop activity, and tired that meant low blood sugar. It was tricky. I could not just lie down and risk going to sleep when I felt tired. I had to check my urine first. This was one time I wanted to see one plus instead of negative. Negative told me nothing. I could be negative in a normal blood sugar range or negative in a hypoglycemic range. Self blood glucose monitoring was not available until after I graduated from college, so I created colors with my urine and made a lot of assumptions.

I made sure my purse with its stash of emergency candy was always nearby before going to sleep. Sometimes I slept on top of it, because as I mentioned, girls were renowned for playing stupid tricks on people who fell asleep. There could not be a trick stupider than taking my candy, but trying to adequately explain that was hard. I imagined the conversation:

Setting: Girls gathered around me listening in rapt attention (which would be the Alpha Miracle in itself...)

Me: "Friends, as some of you know, I have diabetes. That means I have to have candy near me at all...and I mean *all* times, in case my blood sugar gets too low."

Friend: "What is blood sugar?"

Me: "It's sugar in your blood. It has to be at a certain level to function normally. When you have diabetes, your pancreas, which makes insulin, doesn't work right, so your blood sugar can get too high or low."

Friend (puzzled and saddened look on her face): "What does that have to do with not sharing your candy with all of us who are your friends?"

Me: (Sigh) "I don't mean to not share my candy. It's just that if it's gone and my blood sugar gets low I could have a seizure."

(Friends back away with looks of shock and horror.)

Epilogue: I become virtually unclean among my peers, and indeed, never have a lasting friendship of any type and live my life as a hermit on a lone mountain top.

Curtain Falls

The next tricky part was breakfast the morning after our party. Moms often wanted to make what they considered a "treat breakfast" for their daughter and her friends. This usually meant pancakes with a lot of syrup or huge home made cinnamon rolls: hard options for me. Another difficulty was the fact that I needed to take my morning insulin a half hour before we ate. All the other girls got up and stumbled immediately into the kitchen for food. I had to wake up before the others to get my shot or ask the mother to stall breakfast. Sometimes my mom would discuss this with the hostess Mom ahead of time, so she would wake me up quietly before waking the other girls. Occasionally it worked; often it didn't. There was a tremendous amount of playing it by ear, and at times I was tone deaf.

The drama continued with junior high dances. As if these parties were not difficult enough by the mere fact of being an initiation into guy/girl interactions, in addition I had to monitor my food intake and be sure it coincided with my increased activity on the dance floor.

And sometimes off the dance floor. The good thing was that Mom let me go without Horace for dances, so I took in as many as I could.

As I look back now, I realize only the energy of a teenager could withstand such pressure. I was compelled to look normal. Regardless of what normal was, I knew for certain I was not-normal, so the look required a lot of doing. I took playing-it-cool to a new level. My friends thought I was the most in-control person they knew, and I was their confidante. I adopted the teenage facade of immortality and invincibility, thinking I was tremendously in-control as well. Dr. Jackson's statement about being able to do anything anyone else did, often replayed in my mind, while the price, which he had barely alluded to, crystallized.

On the other hand, what I know now, is that I need not have expended so much energy looking in-control. My life would have been easier had I just gone with the flow, asked for help, and let myself mess up occasionally. But messing up was outside my parameters. Kids today seem better at that. I'm proud of them.

Lessons Learned:
1. Despite all my efforts to look normal, between diabetes and Horace, deep inside I knew I was a Freak.
2. Being "normal" has a high price tag.
3. I still don't know why I got diabetes, but I wonder if it might be here to help me...no...that can't be.

CHAPTER 17

Being a Freak loses shock-value with prolonged exposure. In eighth grade diabetes management around basketball was on the downhill slope of the learning curve, I wore Horace after school and during the night, and at least having braces was acceptable, as several of my friends had gotten them. Life was getting easier and I had high hopes. What I did not know was the light at the end of the tunnel was really the oncoming Silver Bullet Express on its way to Abilene.

Nineteen-seventy was a year of demarcation: I graduated from eighth grade, the end of childhood schooling. It also was the year my life changed forever. Again.

Mom and I had driven to Columbia for my usual scoliosis check and x-rays. It had been a long trip and we were tired. It was January and the days were short, dark and cold. We arrived home after dinner-time, but had not yet eaten. As we walked into the house Dad met us in the kitchen.

"You haven't been listening to the radio, have you?

"No. Why?" Mom looked puzzled.

"Come on in, there's something we all need to sit down and talk about."

It sounded ominous. Mom and I walked into the living room where Holly and Janis were already gathered. I sat on a metal desk chair near Janis. Mom sat in the soft red chair, and Dad pulled in a kitchen chair. We huddled, awaiting the Unknown.

Dad cleared his throat. "I didn't want you to hear this on the radio. We got word from Aunt Dorene and Uncle Sydney that Tommy has been killed in action in Vietnam." Dad's voice died in his throat.

Silence pounded my ear drums, relieved rhythmically by the ticking clock. I looked at Janis. Tears streamed down her face, even though she was a senior in high school, nearly a grown-up. I looked at Holly. He was just a sixth grader, so I wasn't surprised to see that tears encircled his eyes but had not yet fallen. Mom sobbed quietly. I looked at Dad: his face was white, his hands clenching into fists and unclenching as if to the beat of his heart. This could not be true.

I moved from a pain-filled multi-dimensional world to a single plane. Cousin Tommy of The Grandiose Event, could not and would not be dead. Not in my world.

Tommy had not wanted to go to Vietnam, but he would not run away either. His draft number was low, too low for us to believe he would escape. We were right, and on June seventeenth, Janis' seventeenth birthday, he left for Basic Training at Fort Leonard Wood, Missouri.

Tommy had spent his life hunting, fishing, and loving the outdoors. He was familiar with guns, but he could not shoot another human being, so he requested the Medic Corp. Surprisingly enough his request was granted. He shipped to Vietnam in November 1969, leaving behind his young wife Judy, and Brandon, their new baby son.

It was an odd thing when he left - he did not think he would come home alive. That fog settled on all of us. Shortly after he was drafted he told my aunt and uncle that when he died he wanted to be buried near the big oak tree at Edinburg Cemetery. The cemetery tucked in beside the country church all of us had attended throughout our childhood, and where many of our ancestors were buried. It was surrounded by deep green woods that Tommy had claimed as his own.

Now it had come home to roost. Two weeks passed before Tommy arrived home...to the funeral home. For Mom the weeks were eternal. For me, it gave more time to pretend nothing had happened.

As we walked into the funeral home, frostbite stabbed to the marrow of my bones. Our family was ushered into a private room where people spoke in hushed tones, deepening the isolation in my world. Uncle Sydney requested the casket be opened, and we walked by single file, gazing into the box.

The still figure did not look much like Tommy...just enough to know it was. He was deeply sun tanned, and badly swollen. His usually lean face puffed out. The funeral director mumbled about the heat in Vietnam making it difficult to preserve a body. Right: this was not Tommy, it was a preserved body.

As I walked from the casket, terror rose in my chest. Fight as I could, I was not able to breathe. I left the room and walked the hallway, gasping for air. As a small child I had asthma so bad, one winter the doctor told my parents to leave for Arizona or I would not make it to spring. We had packed up and left. I got better, and in nine months we came back to Memphis. I rarely thought of asthma attacks anymore. Apparently asthma had waited for me, lurking in the one dimensional world.

The day of the funeral we all dressed as nicely as we could, but with much thought to staying warm at the gravesite. January in Missouri is not a time to be long outdoors dressed in your flimsy Sunday best. At church the casket was parked in front of the pulpit with an American flag draped over it. I had never before thought the flag was ugly.

The sermon was long. Or short? I can't tell you.

Our usual drive to Edinburg took fifteen minutes; ten minutes if Dad drove. Today it took several lifetimes. I was breathing better, but my stomach churned and my head felt close to explosion. We parked, we got out, and we walked to a hole in the ground with a casket suspended over it. Words were said, people cried, and then came time for the twenty-one gun salute.

Army personnel with rifles stood in the woods behind Edinburg. Tommy's woods. Why did they invade it? The commander signaled, guns fired, shots echoed. I clutched my chest. Guns cracked again. No blood came out, but I was sure they had hit me. The one dimension of my world split from the top down, and I was exposed. I stood in the gray arctic beside a sealed casket that held the shell of what used to be Tommy. Cousin Tommy of the Grandiose Event, that would never happen again. I stumbled to the car and collapsed in the back seat.

When the roaring guns stilled, we went to Granny's house. In many ways it was like our traditional Thanksgiving or Christmas gatherings, though the one difference was palpable. If no one spoke to me I could grip my shreds together; if I was called on to speak I dissembled.

No one else cried; I was the oddball. Since the strong charade of Thanksgiving was in progress, when I faltered I bolted for the bathroom. I spoke harshly to myself: *Get a grip! Don't be such a crybaby. Stop being so dramatic; just trying to get attention!* Whose voice was that?

It was a mean trick, and did not stop my crying. Daddy came into the room on one of my crying fits and held me. Once it passed I wiped my red eyes, and took a peek at him. He looked profoundly miserable, but far above crying. It was obvious, to be an adult I needed to get over this crying business.

Several years later, then-President Nixon declared the "dispute" in Vietnam "officially over". I was baby-sitting for one of my favorite families, and had put the children to bed, wanting to be alone when the broadcast aired. As Nixon spoke I sat glued to the television, listening so hard my head ached. Then he said it, "The military action in Vietnam is over."

I stood up transfixed. I flew back to my one dimension world, and here the war raged on. It was not a dispute or military action, it was death, mayhem and destruction. Missiles screamed, bombs exploded, choppers chopped. Tommy lay dead on a battlefield, surrounded by enemy fire. Though it might save other Tommys, this was too little, too late.

In 2002 an *incredible* thing happened. The army called my aunt and uncle, and said they were building a new hospital facility in Fort Hood, Texas. It was to be the newest and largest health clinic in the United States Army, and...would be named after Tommy. Thirty-two years after his death, such a thing.

I learned that such an honor is usually reserved for generals and congressmen, rarely ever an enlisted man. To say I was dumbfounded is to call the Grand Canyon an impressive ditch.

Not being familiar with armed services, I began to hear and piece together the history I had lived through. I knew that after Tommy's death Judy had been given Tommy's medals of award posthumously. I had no idea what they were or what they meant. They did not bring Tommy back, so in my world they were irrelevant. I found out however, that some of them included the Distinguished Service Cross, the Bronze Star, and the Air Medal. The Distinguished Service Cross is the second highest award for valor by a soldier.

I remembered that in Tommy's death, lives had been saved, but in 1970 I was in no condition to take in the whole story. In 2002, I read the account of his bravery, and have recounted it below. I am filled with awe and sadness.

"For extraordinary heroism in action, Private First Class Charles T. Moore, United States Army, distinguished himself by extraordinary heroism in action on 5 January 1970, in the Republic of Vietnam.

On that date, when the First Platoon of Company D made contact with a determined enemy force located in a well-fortified bunker complex, a friendly trooper to the front was severely wounded.

Despite his own wrist wounds, Private Moore, medical aidman for the First Platoon, moved through the intense hail of enemy fire to treat and evacuate the wounded soldier.

Subsequently, a rocket impacted which strafed the area with shrapnel, wounding the First Platoon leader and further injuring Private Moore. Again, with complete disregard for his own welfare, private Moore moved to the aid of his platoon leader and evacuated the officer to safety.

Then, noticing that his first patient had stopped breathing, Private Moore untiringly, and singularly performed mouth-to-mouth resuscitation until life and unassisted breathing were restored.

As he was constructing a bamboo stretcher on which to carry this critically wounded trooper, Private Moore was shot in the hip and rendered unconscious.

Minutes later, he regained consciousness, and although his many wounds now completely incapacitated his movement and his position was exposed, he began shouting valuable instructions concerning the necessary and vital treatment for the wounded.

Even when he knew death was imminent, Private Moore unselfishly ignored his pain and continued to give valuable medical instructions.

Private Moore succumbed to his wounds before he could be medically evacuated, but not before he had saved the lives of many of his comrades through his conspicuous gallantry and extraordinary heroism."

Tommy was killed in Vietnam. You might think over the years the blow has softened, and wars of today make more sense than the insanity of the war in Vietnam. You would be wrong.

Crusades that explode into military action, even today, are making less and less sense. The fierce need for greed, control and superiority, backed by a strong political good ol' boys club, slices through as a resilient causative factor. Young men with more energy than wisdom, dance as pawns for older, yet equally unconscious men, to the tune of *War is the Answer.* If it is, so what on earth is the question?

Lessons Learned:

1. Pretending it isn't so prolongs the inevitable. But sometimes it is a necessary reprieve.
2. If you hear a twenty-one gun salute in preparation, run like all hell is behind you.
3. None of us gets off this planet alive, but I wish some of us could have stayed longer.
4. At the end of the game, both pawns and kings all go back in the same box.

CHAPTER 18

I was finally there: a sophomore. No longer a freshman, no longer in junior high. I had arrived, traversing a vast and tumultuous journey that in my estimation, made crossing the Rockies in a Conestoga wagon a mundane effort.

I was now old enough to go on an actual date...yet one more new conundrum. Although dating is a conundrum for all of us in the beginning, I had lots of extra things to think about. Especially considering my zeal to look normal which, at a subterranean level, had become my new religion. The abnormal effort I put into looking normal was astounding.

If I went for a dinner date, which at fifteen rarely happened, how would I inconspicuously take my shot before eating? The easy answer was to put my insulin and syringe in my purse, excuse myself to go to the restroom after ordering my food, and shoot up. Then return to my date, as if I had needed to powder my nose.

That was all fine and good on formal dinner dates, but what about hayrides accompanied by a campfire and wienie roast? That was more difficult. For one thing, nobody took a purse on a hayride/wienie roast for heaven's sake. So...what to do?

At that time (post-sock hop, but pre-Reagan years) people did not carry fanny packs. Things are much easier today. Back then I shoved my insulin vials and syringe in the back pocket of my bell bottoms. That worked fine until my date worked up enough courage to explore feminine topography below the equator. At that point he discovered two hard lumps and a syringe.

The syringe was hardest to explain. Back then people were very, *very* uptight about syringes. Especially on a church sponsored hayride and campfire. It is a wonder I was not arrested or burned in the campfire as an infidel.

Relief came once I dated a guy long enough to feel comfortable telling him about my diabetes. That usually took three or four dates. There obviously were different reactions. Sometimes the guy would be totally freaked out by the fact that I had to give myself shots several times a day. With those guys, I did not *even* discuss urine testing, and they rarely lasted long. Diabetes was a good test of character.

Other guys however, showed more promise, being at ease with the idea. One guy even asked if he could give my shot. He was less interested when I let him do it in my arm instead of my hip. I gleaned an early understanding of men that takes some women years of listening to country music to discover.

Then there was Prom Night. When I was a sophomore, I was asked to the Junior-Senior Prom by an upperclassman. That fell well within the Dreams and Fantasies section of my diary, but far outside my Perception of Reality. What a rush!

However, back to the overall life considerations incurred by diabetes. Prom Night *is not* just an evening affair. It lasts from early evening on Prom Night, through the night and into the next morning, so the insulin thing was tricky.

While other girls were concentrating on the right dress, right shoes, perfect manicure and pedicure, latest and greatest hairstyling, most alluring perfume, right underwear...I was trying to figure out which insulin to inject, at what time, and how to know when I might need more insulin or more food. Then there was the question of how to shove my insulin syringe, urine test equipment and food supply into one of those sequined evening bags the size of a brussel sprout. As if that was not enough, did I mention, the guy was from out of town, so I would stay with his parents for the weekend? Dear God...

I decided to treat it like a Slumber Party. You might imagine I did not share that simile with my mother. In my favor was that I knew the guy well enough to tell him I had diabetes. That opened the way for discussion, and kept me from using a ton of energy trying to be covert about what I needed to do for myself. He was clueless however, about all it *really* meant.

He understood I had to take a shot before we had dinner, again before breakfast, and I would need to have food or candy with me at all times.

That was a good start. He put candy in his tuxedo pocket and snack crackers in the car glove box. I found it very endearing. Dating with diabetes brought out a different kind of attractiveness in men.

I toiled over how much to teach him versus how much time I really had to do it. After all, this had taken me three years of intense personal learning, plus more than my lifetime of vicarious learning from Janis. There was the issue of being nervous and losing my appetite at dinner which could result in low blood sugar. Or my nervousness could trigger an adrenalin response resulting in high blood sugar. Then there was the issue of dancing for hours and hours, and what that does to blood sugar. There was an additional issue of simply being awake all night and moving around instead of sleeping, which can lead to low blood sugar all on its own. There was of course, the issue of eating breakfast at three in the morning instead of the usual six a.m. There was the alcohol issue, and last, but certainly not least was the issue of making out all night, which opens another entire series of didactic lectures. These things had an effect on blood sugar not only during Prom Night, but for the next twenty-four hours after as well, and I will not even *touch* the potential long-range effects of making out all night. I doubted he was up for that much education. I would have to play it by ear, and he would just have to let me lead.

Leaving town for the weekend for this event meant my parents and I were taking a huge leap of faith. HUGE! Immense. Gargantuan. I am immensely proud of my parents for trusting me. If I had a child and was in the same circumstance, I hope I would trust as they did, but I wouldn't bet on it. On Prom night I'm guessing they slept less than I did.

It all worked out, and I am here to write about it. However, there was one precarious situation that evening worth elaboration. I had adorned myself exquisitely, and looked, in my estimation, like a Royal Goddess. It had taken hours of shopping, bathing, plucking, shaving, oiling, perfuming, painting, coiffing and dressing. No small task. Then we went to dinner. I excused myself after ordering and went to shoot up in the restroom. He gave me a reassuring wink as I left, letting me know he knew what was going on, so I felt like we were somewhat in this together. At the Prom we danced divinely, chatted with friends, and danced some more. Whenever

I felt my blood sugar dropping I drank punch or ate snacks. So far, so good.

Next was the After-Prom party. This was a hayride sponsored by his church. (Hayrides in my part of the country – the Midwest - were ubiquitous; more plentiful than the McDonald's that were beginning to sweep the land.) Seemingly simple enough, however the guys smuggled a significant amount of alcohol onto the wagon and got progressively relaxed-yet-amorous as the hayride ensued. No problem...I still was in control. I had my insulin in one jeans pocket and candy in the other.

Until the cap came off my syringe which then stabbed me in the keister.

At first I thought it was a splinter from the hay wagon, but facts became apparent. I coyly tried to pull the syringe out of my jeans, but it was wedged. Imagine those Super Glue commercials where they pick up a semi tractor-trailer with a crane that is adhered via the mega-glue.

After several attempts, I finally had to ask my boyfriend for assistance. He was more than eager to assist with anything having to do with close proximity to my derrière, and for a period of time, I am pretty sure he was trying to extricate the paraphernalia with his mouth. Not highly efficient, but pleasurable.

He finally got the syringe out and gallantly kissed my owie. His lips slowly tiptoed up my back, then hesitated, nuzzling the back of my neck. It did remove all thought of pain from my stab wound. There were some good things about having diabetes.

After the hayride and syringe-in-keister experience, excitement was running high. We went to his car, and of course parked along a country road. What else was there to do in rural Americana in the early 1970's? People were not yet into getting hotel rooms after Prom; we went out to "hear the corn breathe". That was the line. I am not sure how many girls actually believed it, but it was more than moderately effective, considering the number of cars parked along this particular road. This corn must have been doing jumping jacks.

My candy supply had dwindled to a miniscule two pieces and the snack crackers were history. I was having an exceptionally difficult time trying to decide the source of my adrenalin rush. Was it from low blood sugar...or did I just really have the hots for this guy? Stopping the action for a false alarm seemed like a waste of adrenalin. What to do?

I decided sooner or later, if it was low blood sugar I would get weak and shaky, my clue to eat the candy. Within ten minutes my adrenalin rush was over, and what was happening in the back seat of his silver Camero did not hold my interest. Darn. I ate the candy and we headed to his house for snacks. Ah....growing up with diabetes.

By the time I reached my junior year in high school, I had figured out most conundrums, with a plan for each. Or so I thought. The spring of that year my usual allergies became worse than usual. I was miserable, and of course I shared my misery with my mother. She called our family doctor (not our diabetes doctor), asking if there wasn't something that might be done to relieve my never-ending wheezing, coughing, sniffling, sneezing, choking allergic symptoms.

Kindly, he assured her there was. He prescribed a packet of pills for me. One was to be taken each day for twenty days. He explained they started with a low dosage and worked to a higher dosage, thereafter they would decrease in dose again, at which time I would probably be nearly symptom free. I was thrilled! I gulped the first pill before leaving the pharmacy.

On the third day of pills my urine test before breakfast was negative, but before lunch it was four plus. I was puzzled. I ate half my lunch, thinking that would have me back to negative before dinner. I was wrong. My test was still four plus, I was irritated, and the fact that I was hungry as a bear did not help matters.

I took one extra unit of Regular insulin (the only fast-acting insulin available back then) before dinner, and ate only my protein exchanges. By bedtime my urine test was down to one percent. *What?!* Things were headed in the right direction, but my efforts were greatly under-rewarded. I racked my brain for what was wrong. Was I getting sick, but didn't feel it yet? Was I nervous about something? I couldn't come up with an answer, but high blood sugar always handed my internal-accuser ammunition for a guilty-until-proven-innocent verdict.

The next morning my test was negative. I breathed a sigh of relief and went to school thinking whatever "it" was, now was not. Before lunch my urine test was negative again. However, before dinner, that nasty orange color reared its ugly head: four plus. I did a "double void", meaning that after my first test I drank several glasses of water and retested my urine in twenty minutes. I also did a more diluted test that measured higher than four plus. My urine measured five percent glucose.

There was no reason for this! I had followed all the (bad word) rules. I showed Mom and we discussed what I ate for lunch. Nothing added up. I self-induced a fast until my urine test was negative (passive resistance, similar to a sit-in, which was becoming popular). Mom was not in favor of my Ghandi behavior, but was too wise to intervene. I drank glass after glass of water, trying to dilute and pee out my sugar, and ran up and down our sixteen-step staircase fifty-two times. I was trying for sixty, but wore out. By bedtime I was back down to two plus, a sniveling trifle compared to all my efforts.

The next morning I woke up dreading my urine test. I did a double void, knowing the first one would still hold sugar from the night before. It was negative. I was relieved, but wary. Before lunch I tested my urine – two plus. What was going on? I ate no lunch at all and did a double void before dinner – five percent! I was beside myself. After a week of this I had lost five pounds, which was a nice benefit, but my urine tests were consistently going higher. Finally, Mom and I caught on. We called the doctor who had prescribed the allergy pills. You already may have guessed what they were...prednisone. A steroid.

Yes, the good news is they helped decrease my allergies significantly. The bad news is if I had continued to take them, I may have ended up in a coma from diabetic ketoacidosis...in addition to starving!

How did I feel about this little event? Horribler than horrible. I felt betrayed. Neurotic perfectionism about my diabetes had been honed to a fine science, yet I was completely out of control. Nothing I had been taught helped me overcome the Enemy.How did my doctor react when my mother asked him about the medication?

"Oh, I forgot she has diabetes. Yes, the medication could be causing her blood sugar to go up, but it shouldn't be serious."

WHAAAAAAAAATTT? Not serious...????? Perhaps I over-reacted, but I wanted to grab the man by his necktie, swing him around the room a few dozen times and release his hulk into a brick wall. I had starved for over a week trying to get a grip on my glucose levels, because he *forgot* I had diabetes. Why didn't he just *ask?* Now there's a thought.

It was a lesson I did not forget. Having diabetes means I have to know as much as I possibly can about everything going on with, or going into, my body. I have to ask all the right questions, and anticipate a few others, just in case the health care provider does not think to ask me the right question. Succinctly, I have to become mildly-to-moderately paranoid about my own self-care. I wonder if this was a turning point for me in knowing I had no other career choice than health care. My only defense was a good offense.

Lessons Learned:
1. Telling a guy I had diabetes could often sort the keepers from the throw-backs.
2. Amorous excitement can mimic the jitters of low blood sugar. Most often, I did not share this fact with boyfriends.
3. Statistically, doctors are more fallible than parachutes.

CHAPTER 19

As I neared college, new considerations came to my horizon. In the realm of dating, I began to look at guys differently. Solid, dependable and smart started ranking as high as good-looking. I was uncertain about having children, as health risks for a pregnant diabetic woman and her unborn child in 1973 were significant. Blood glucose monitoring was still done via the unreliable surrogate of urine testing. I found myself focusing more on whether or not someone I dated would be a good lifetime partner; it was a little shocking. Besides all that, I was very serious about college, and planned to go into medicine, so academics was my conscious and verbally-stated priority. On a subconscious and hormonal level, other priorities may have been in play. The beauty of youth is that it allows enough energy to sustain both.

College was my first trial at taking complete care of myself. I was fortunate Mom taught me to enjoy all sorts of foods, because that is what was available at college. Some sorts shared a greater resemblance to items found in a back alley trash can than a café table. The lettuce usually looked like it had been through the dishwasher before being served. What they tried to pass off as hamburger was truly an alien meat. Having grown up on a farm, I was accustomed to eating beef from our stock of certified Angus cattle. I was astounded by the packing peanuts someone had ground and dyed a mysterious brown, labeling it "hamburger". I knew better. But I ate it, and counted it as two meat exchanges.

Other foods were trickier, like the stuff they called goulash. I had trouble identifying the amount of meat it contained, (Was there really meat or were those large pepper flakes?) and trying to figure out how much pasta (bread exchange) and olive oil (fat exchange) was nearly impossible. Fortunately Mom and Dad had gotten a small refrigerator for my room, which required special permission from the Dean (...how times have changed...), for cheese, milk, fruit and other healthier and less mysterious snacks.

No one was available to help me give injections in those hard-to-reach places, so I did what I could to continue rotating injection sites. Sometimes it was challenging, sometimes it was painful, and sometimes I just did not rotate. So shoot me...preferably in a hard-to-reach place, if you don't mind.

Remembering to do my urine tests was not a problem; I still lived and died by being negative. It was like clockwork: I got up, did my test and shot, then the day started. Between classes and lunch I peed on test tape that I kept in my purse, and headed to the cafeteria. Test tape was a Godsend. It still consisted of turning your pee vibrant colors, but all I had to do was tear off a strip, pee on it, and wait one minute for it to turn a color. My diabetes health care professionals told me it was less accurate than testing with the kit, but let me tell you, it won hands down in the fitting-in-your-purse category. Before dinner, I tested and shot up, and last thing before going to bed I did my test, washed my face and brushed my teeth. It did not matter what time it was or where I was; by this time being obsessive-compulsive had integrated into my DNA.

Janis and I had our final Gifford Sisters visit to the diabetes clinic shortly before I went to college. In my ongoing effort to escape home, I finished high school a semester early, so I was seventeen. Janis was twenty-one, and working on her first degree, which was in journalism. Her second degree was in nursing, but I digress.

Obviously, we were far from the Pediatric age group, but upon Mom and Dad's request, Dr. Jackson still saw us. We did not know of an adult diabetes specialist, and going to an unknown physician gave us concern (read: scared us into Pampers). At this last visit we saw Dr. Richard Guthrie, who had worked with Dr. Jackson for several years. He and his wife, Diana, were leaving the University to start a diabetes practice together in Wichita, Kansas. Diana was a Diabetes Nurse Specialist, and their practice would work with both adult and pediatric diabetic patients. I wished they were moving close enough for me to see them for diabetes care, but no such luck. However, as synchronicity would have it, our paths would cross again.

College years brought more surprises than I had expected. In my first year of college, I met someone who made marriage seem like a good idea. Let me explain my preconceived notions on marriage. Prior to leaving for college I had cemented the idea that I would go to college, then medical school, and finally residency and possibly do a fellowship. After completing those ten to fifteen years I would start practice, and when I had enough money to buy my own house that had a swimming pool in the living room, *then* I would find a husband and get married. Ideas such as this grow like unruly weeds when you are a thinker.

The idea of going through medical school as a married female student did not feel right for me. I didn't think I could juggle the demands of both. This was the early 1970s, and although the women's movement was gearing up, I grew up in a conservative rural town, attending three church services each week as well as choir practice, in the most conservative church in that conservative town, AND I attended college at that church's institution of higher learning. Some of the education was so heavenly, it was of no earthly good.

I was accepted to a six year medical program at the University of Missouri in Kansas City, but their schedule required I start in mid-semester the following year. Waiting has never been my strong point.

I had things to do, places to go, people to see. Also, the thought of constant school, year-round, with the intensity required by a medical program began to seem like an artificially induced incarceration. I was unconvinced of the wisdom of this tightly defined box, and considering my experience with medical personnel; even more ponderous about who I might be once they released me upon the world.

I took a battery of guidance tests that helped students find careers most fitting with their personalities, likes and dislikes. I was certain my test would say "Impending Physician"; I was wrong. The report said my preferences fit more in line with nursing or teaching, than medicine.

Whoever created this test obviously was in dire error. Medicine would be my life. I had been on a one-track path for med school since seventh grade. I had taken every science and math course available and nearly killed myself to maintain a 3.95 GPA. I *was* going to med school!

Maybe.

My heart stubbornly interrupted my brilliance. It was a very trying time, to say the least, and maybe one I'll share in another book, but for now, (I'll try to stay on track) let me simply say in 1975 I decided to go into nursing. And I got married. A decision for which I have long been grateful. (The nursing, not the marriage.) However, nursing had its problematic issues as well.

The nursing school I attended was in the midst of its own Civil War, with one of the Underling Instructors openly challenging the Chairperson for her position. You might imagine that strife trickled down to us peons, the students. You would be right. I held a firm belief that has strengthened over time: Nursing is a profession that eats its young.

Medicine, on the other hand takes a more masculine approach. They use sleep deprivation and long hours of overwork during the internship and residency years. These two tools, well-known to schools of brainwashing tactics, such as prisons and military boot camp, rip down the individual so he can be rebuilt in the gleaming image of his Teacher. Such rebuilding grants him (and sometimes her) the privilege of entering at the Sacred Doors of the Medical Machine.

Though this process is effective in cloning replicas, sometimes the Rebuilt One retains remnants of his/her soul. Or, over time, they grow a new one. Regardless, none pass through the Holy Halls unscathed.

Yes, nursing school held surprises. I discovered there was no nursing subspecialty for diabetes! In my sophomore year I discussed with my advisor that I wanted to go into nursing to help people with diabetes. She said, "Well, do you prefer medical-surgical or pediatrics?"

I paused, thinking she misunderstood. "I want to help people with diabetes. I want to do diabetes education." I spoke slowly and enunciated clearly.

"Rachel, there is no nursing specialty in diabetes. Do you want to work with children or adults with diabetes?"

"Yes."

"Yes...which?" Her tone hinted of dwindling patience.

"Yes, I want to work with all people who have diabetes."

Her tone wasn't hinting anymore, "That's not our system."

I paused. "Then I need to think about it."

Clinical rotations began, and I liked medical – surgical (med-surg) nursing okay, but it lit no fires under me. Then I did obstetrics/gynecology. That was a happenin' place. Exciting things were popping right and left – literally. People were screaming, patients were speed-raced into the Delivery Room, and brand new lives entered the world. Wow.

Then I did pediatrics. The first time I saw a tiny power-packed five-year-old boy grab his IV pole and sprint to the playroom dragging the pole behind him (the day after his hernia operation) - I knew I had found my home. Kids were hysterical, fun, totally honest...and they got well fast! Life was everywhere. I jumped in head-first.

Lessons Learned:
1. College is an intense time of growing up, just like learning to walk is. The number of times you topple over is similar, too.
2. It would be a good thing to create a university that provides true education without all the Ivory Towering.

PART THREE:

THE JOURNEY CONTINUES

Chapter 20

My first year of actual nursing in 1979, was nothing less than harrowing. Between graduating from college and starting my real job at Kansas University Medical Center, affectionately called KUMC for obvious reasons, I enthusiastically volunteered to be nurse at the local diabetes camp. Only the wild enthusiasm and naiveté of youth could have prompted me to do such a thing. My husband was not thrilled to have me gone for ten days, but I'm sorry to say there was little he was happy about at that time.

Camp was ten days long, in the middle of hot, steamy July, in a park from where it was soon moved due to an escalating crime rate. That's the good part.

I, as a twenty-three year old graduate nurse (did not even have my license yet), was the only nurse in the camp of fifty-two children. The camp physician came to camp for dinner, and we met to discuss appropriate insulin and food changes for the campers. Then he left. Dear God...what was I thinking?

During the day, camp was nonstop activity: swimming, horseback riding, hiking, running, you name it. At home these children never exercised this much, so as you might guess, their blood sugars fell through the floor. The first night I did cabin rounds at midnight, and gave nine injections of Glucagon (a shot that raises blood sugar when a diabetic person is too unconscious to eat). I got done at three-ten a.m.; ten minutes late for starting my three o'clock rounds. It went downhill from there. I gave another fifteen injections of Glucagon that night, sprinting through the thick black woods, from cabin to cabin, like a rabbit with its tail on fire.

When the physician arrived that following evening, we dropped *everybody's* insulin. That night I gave only five Glucagon injections. By the third night I thought I might get a few hours of sleep. I was wrong.

Just as I finished midnight rounds around two-thirty a.m. a carload of exceptionally drunk young men drove up the steep winding gravel camp path to my front door – literally. Up, over the steps of my cabin, onto the concrete landing, with the grill shoving a pregnant profile into my screen door. I had no inside door.

I did what any wisdom-filled twenty-two year old sleep-deprived woman would do. I screamed, "GET OFF MY PORCH!" slammed the door to my boudoir, and fell into bed. Not sure when they left, but they were gone by reveille.

My job at KUMC started four days after camp. On my first day, the head nurse informed me that everyone working at the Medical Center did rotating shifts. For those who have never done rotating shifts, let me explain. Hospitals are a twenty-four hour business, so somebody has to be working all the time. At our hospital, day shift started at seven a.m. and stopped at three-thirty p.m. Evening shift started at three p.m. and stopped at eleven-thirty p.m., and night shift was from eleven p.m. to seven-thirty a.m. Rotating shifts meant you had to rotate sequentially through all three shifts. I was not pleased.

In college, I had worked the night shift at a food manufacturing plant. The life of a nocturnal animal gave me the demeanor of a vampire. I could not imagine getting used to the constant upheaval of changing from a vampire to an early bird. It would be hard to switch my insulin regimen around, too, but I figured I could if I had to. Never, in all my life, had I used diabetes as an excuse to get out of anything...until then. I told my head nurse I could rotate between day and evening shifts, but I could not do night shifts because of my diabetes. I tried to look forthright and nonchalant when I said it, but a voice in my head screamed, "You faker! Shirk! Weenie!!"

Fortunately, she did not hear that voice. It was written into my contract that night shifts would be omitted from my scheduling. I was ecstatic. I also was dumbfounded; diabetes had actually worked in my favor.

During my first year working the Pediatric unit and Pediatric Intensive Care I told my head nurse I wanted to work with children who had diabetes, so whenever a diabetic child came on the unit I was assigned to him or her. It was wonderful! My own diabetes hospital stay (what you waded through in Section One) was as vivid for me then as it probably is for you right now. I wanted so much to make the hospitalization for these children less painful, more comforting, and definitely kinder and gentler. As soon as I met the children I let them know I had diabetes, and that it takes a lot of learning, but I knew they could do it. I passed on the hope Dr. Jackson had given me as often as I could. I often found myself crying with these children. In nursing school I was taught such behavior was the epitome of unprofessionalism, but I could not help it. When they cried, I held their hands, and we cried together.

On one occasion my little ten-year-old girl patient Lindsey, and her family, were gathered so I could teach them insulin injection. Everyone was in anxious attendance: Mom, Dad, little brother, and Lindsey. I let Lindsey draw up sterile saline as though it were insulin. Then I let her give me a shot in the arm. I can't say I was not a little worried.

I anticipated it might be more painful than when I injected myself, but when she wound up like a pitcher for the Yankees, and slammed the needle into my arm, I almost went into shock. Her family clapped and cheered, furthering the ballpark ambiance.

"You said the quicker I went through the skin, the less it would hurt. Did it hurt?" She looked up at me with the eyes of an angel.

I lied. "No...uh...no, not at all." My voice resonated with surprising strength.

Then she drew up her injection, and gave it in her leg. As she removed the needle, we were in awe. Tears flowed like champagne at a wedding party; it was an amazing moment.

I loved pediatrics and I loved my patients, but a gentle nudge in my heart made me impatient. I needed to do the next thing...if only I knew what that was.

I started to check around with diabetes education centers in the city. Everyone seemed to want someone with prior experience. It astounded me that living with diabetes for more than a decade did not qualify as experience. What school did *they* go to?

I checked with my head nurse to see if she had any ideas.

She did. She recommended talking to the Head of Pediatric Endocrinology at our Medical Center.

Why didn't I think of that?!

I stealthily watched for the Head of Pediatric Endocrinology, I'll call him Dr. Brain, to come to the Peds ICU where I was working. I did not leave for lunch, being afraid I would miss him. My nerves were on edge. Why on earth would he want to hire *me*? I had only one year of nursing experience. I had only a Bachelor's degree. I wasn't even sure he knew my name.

He came into the unit followed, as always, by six or eight worried-looking young people in white coats. Most of them I knew, but on occasion I wondered if a local vagrant might have gotten caught up in the parade.

It would be easier to talk to Dr. Brain about a job opportunity had he been doing rounds alone. My heart skipped several beats and my throat went dry. However, I was in charge of the ICU that day, so eventually he would have to talk to me, even if only to ask for a chart. I bided my time...for about ten seconds. My patience ran out with a loud bang that impelled me toward him like an Olympic starting gun.

"Dr. Brain, how are you today?"

He glanced my way. "Um hmm." Dr. Brain was not known for being chatty.

"Uh...when you're done with rounds could I speak with you for a moment?"

He already had looked away from me (did he ever really *look* at me?), and his body language made it clear he was unaware I existed. He mumbled toward the wall, "...just talk now."

Darn! I did not want to blabber on about wanting to work in his clinic when all the stooges were there. What if he laughed at the idea? What if the stooges laughed? How dumb would I feel then? I decided to slow my neurosis from a full gallop to a nominal trot, catch my breath, and just ask.

"I'd like to work with an outpatient diabetes group doing education. I wondered if you might have a position open?" There, I said it. I looked at the floor and tried to calm myself as I waited for his Thanks-but-no-thanks-response. The waiting continued for what seemed like roughly eight days.

"Actually, I need someone right now to run our Biostator® program."

"It's okay, I understand, thank you for..." I suddenly stopped. Although I had no idea what a Biostator® was, it hit me that he might be offering me a job. "Uh...oh...um...what is a Biostator®?"

That is when life dropped in with a beautiful synchronicity. The Pediatric Outpatient Diabetes group needed a nurse to develop and direct a Biostator® (mechanical artificial pancreas) program. In 1982, the Biostator® was very new on the market, so I would be creating a cutting-edge program. The machine continuously withdrew minute amounts of blood, tested the glucose level and responded appropriately with calculated dosages of insulin and/or glucose. It would be used for diabetic patients undergoing surgery or blood glucose re-regulation, and for women during labor and delivery (I remembered my excitement with ob/gyn). It also was used extensively for research protocols. Most of this I learned *after* I accepted the position. Life said, "Looky, an opportunity!" I said, "Yehaaaa!" One of my strong points is enthusiasm; sometimes it works out fine, sometimes it's a lot of work. This was both.

Lessons Learned:

1. "Rotating" and "shifts" are two words that should not be vocalized sequentially.
2. Sometimes being "unprofessional" is not only required, it's the Right thing to be.
3. In the famous words of the prophet Nike: "Just Do It!"

CHAPTER 21

When I started my new job in 1981, the Biostator® was still on back-order. That seemed to be no problem for Dr. Brain, as he put me to work in his lab doing basic science research while we waited for the machine. I thought this would be interesting and good experience. I was right about the latter, but the former lasted about two weeks.

I am not a bench researcher; I am a people-person. Putting aliquot after aliquot of stuff into test tubes for hours at a time became boring very fast. Then my assays didn't work right. My radioimmunoassays (RIA) came back with values all over the place. There was no pattern. Now you might imagine I cleverly knew that meant the assay did not "bind". If so, you would be vastly overestimating my ability at the time.

It took some significant consultation with Dr. Brain before I had any idea what happened. Then it was back to the lab (oh joy, oh ecstasy...) to do it all again. For days. I called the researcher who did the original study I was replicating, and asked for the "cookbook version" of how to do the RIA. I followed the directions to the letter. My RIA still did not bind. I realized research of this type did not stimulate me in the least, and prayed for the Biostator® to arrive.

Then came research with rats. That was a whole new ballgame. My thoughts on rats were that they spread bubonic plague and should be exterminated; I had no other belief about them. However, these rats were white and had big red eyes and soft fur. They looked kind of like tiny kittens, except for their tails: long, skinny and shiny with no fur at all, wherein their cuteness stopped. That, and the fact that they would just as soon sink their teeth into you as look at you, which they did at whim (the sinking, not the looking). However, I am an animal lover, and when it came time to experiment on the rat, I just did not have it in me. In this instance, I think I was a great disappointment to Dr. Brain.

The good news was that the Biostator® finally arrived. The bad news was that it came in several boxes, with "some assembly required".

Dr. Brain pointed me toward the boxes, "There it is. Get it together and working."

I stared dumbly. It did not occur to me he might be serious. The vast majority of my "assembly" knowledge consisted of understanding what a hammer and nail looked like. I also was familiar with screws and the fact that some had a "plus" on the top and some had a "minus", thus requiring a different type of screwdriver for each. I went for a cup of coffee.

On some subconscious level a suspicion floated across the glassy seas of my brain, that Dr. Brain might consider it my job to construct the dismembered Biostator®, regardless of ineptitude. It was not logical, so I left it to drift.

After several days, the boxes remained unopened. I wondered when the assembly people would come to breathe life into the sleeping Biostator® . Later that day I walked into the lab, and Dr. Brain was sitting on the floor, surrounded by blue and silver parts marked "Biostator", with a large manual in one hand and a screwdriver in the other (it was a "plus" screwdriver). That's when my suspicion caught anchor. I quickly ducked out of sight and took several gulps of air. I had to hide out for as long as it took him to provide the assembly required. If he saw me, he might hand me the plus screwdriver.

I fled to the radioactive room and read journal articles until I glowed in the dark. As I suspected, the room was empty. People who are not on the lam are unwilling to risk their gonads to such exposure. I stayed until the fear of sterility and cancer overrode my fear of resurrecting the Biostator® , then moved on to the "cold room" where I created new assays and aliquoted for the rest of the day. When I returned to the scene of the crime, I was thrilled to discover that Dr. Brain had the Biostator® fully assembled, plugged in and humming. Shirking a job was incompatible with my obsessive-compulsive nature, so my relief was palpable.

My ability to operate the Biostator® came with some fear and trembling, but within a short time I was fairly accomplished and able to train a team of nurses as well. We were off and running. We used it for more research than you could shake a proverbial stick (or test tube) at, numerous surgeries, blood glucose re-regulations and I saw many a baby born while their mother and I Biostated together during her labor and delivery. It was fascinating!

But I have gotten ahead of myself. Remember when I said Dr. Guthrie and I would cross paths again? It so happened, that Dr. Guthrie had been using a Biostator® for quite some time in his practice in Wichita, Kansas. His practice was affiliated with Kansas University Medical Center in Kansas City, where our fledgling Biostator® program was located. You guessed it, Dr. Brain knew Dr. Guthrie, so I was sent to Wichita for a week to learn how to operate the Biostator®. For me it was "Old Home Week". For my husband, it was another opportunity to practice his sulking skills, which were already pretty well-honed at this point in our marriage. Suffice it to say things at home were mildly-to-moderately malignant.

Belinda Childs (Lindy) and Kirby Conley were the nurses who operated the Biostator® for Dr. Guthrie, and Lindy kindly invited me to spend the week with her and her husband, staying in their guest bedroom. I accepted their offer, and thus began a long and lovely friendship. Diabetes did a huge favor in guiding me to such good friends.

Lindy, Kirby and Dr. Guthrie took me under their wings, and by the end of the week my proficiency at operating the Biostator® was better than fair-to-partly-cloudy. During that week I was hooked to the machine myself for a period of time, and enjoyed eating ice cream, cake, Twinkies and every other food that raises blood sugar fast and far. Suddenly I was not diabetic anymore. It was like flying, except for the fact that I had IVs in each arm and could not move more than three feet from a machine that stood higher than my waist and had to be pushed around on a cart.

Yet, I was amazed to eat without thinking how much insulin I needed before or afterward. Of course, such eating would have catapulted me into obesity in a heartbeat had I done it all the time, but for the moment it was ecstasy.

Also during that week, I slept with Lindy's dog. This may sound a little kinky, but I assure you it was fairly normal. Lindy and her husband, Rick, had a huge (we are talking HUGE) English Sheepdog named Anastasia, "Annie" for short. I had taken Annie's bed for the week, as she usually slept in the guest bedroom. Lindy warned me about this, telling me to be sure I tightly closed the bedroom door before going to sleep. So I did.

However, that was irrelevant for a hefty sheepdog like Annie. Around midnight I heard the door creak open and before I could realize I might have something to fear, Kerrrrr- *thunk!* Eighty pounds of sheepdog landed on top of me, snuffled me from head to foot, and decided I was inedible, but acceptable. Annie gave me a few slobbery kisses across the forehead and mouth, flopped herself across me, and immediately started snoring.

I was a bit unnerved. As I mentioned however, I am an animal lover, so it worked out fine. The most difficult part was drowning out Annie's snores so I could get back to sleep.

During this visit I also was introduced to what was then called HBGM – or Home Blood Glucose Monitoring, which is now called SBGM (Self Blood Glucose Monitoring). The earliest blood glucose meters were about a foot long, eight inches wide, two or three inches deep, and had to be plugged into a wall socket. The finger stick was done with a metal lancet similar to those used when my brother and I were forced into research at the University of Missouri, so many years ago. They left a slash in your finger instead of a tiny prick. Also, we did not yet realize poking the sides of fingers caused less pain than wounding the fingertip. A large drop of blood was required to cover the early reagent pads; after one minute blood was washed from the pad, which was then blotted and put into the meter for reading. Quite a process.

Those of you who have started doing blood glucose monitoring in the past few years are surely thinking I roamed the plains with the dinosaurs. You also may think doing finger stick blood glucose monitoring is the bane of diabetes existence. Not long ago I heard a television show discussing diabetes, and the statement was made, "Doing a finger stick is awful. It's worse than giving my shots." Well...I have to admit, I come from a different perspective.

As I've mentioned (o'er and o'er again), while growing up with diabetes I did urine tests, which was embarrassing, not terribly helpful, and considered "unclean". It did turn pee interesting colors, so what? It did not give a number, so I could not calculate how much extra insulin or food I needed. In fact, the urine tested was usually several hours old, so sugar that showed up in the urine might not be indicative of the current blood sugar. In that case you had to do a double void, which I mentioned earlier. Sometimes this had to be done during school, which meant a lot of time was lost from class or recess going to the bathroom, testing, drinking water, and starting the whole dreaded process over again. Is blood testing starting to sound better?

Not only that, but when the urine test was negative, there was no way to know if it was negative within a safe range or starting to dip dangerously low. As I look back on those days, I cannot tell you how much I hated urine testing, and how I longed for a way to actually *know* what my blood sugar was, so I could *treat* it instead of playing ring-around-the-rosie.

Back then, the favored tool to decrease elevated blood sugar was to exercise or decrease food intake. What we now know is that exercising with an elevated blood sugar may cause the blood sugar to rise higher. We did not know that then. Yes...we were dinosaurs. To say that I love blood sugar monitoring is an understatement. When I was first able to actually test my own blood sugar and react with one unit of fast-acting insulin for every fifty mg/dl that my blood sugar was above one hundred, I was beyond ecstasy. About a thousand missing puzzle pieces suddenly clicked into place.

During my time in Wichita I also had my first hemoglobin A1c test done. Take a wild guess what it was. Nineteen percent. As you may know, the A1c goal for people with diabetes is less than six-and-a-half to seven percent. Nineteen is equivalent to what I saw in some of our patients who were consistently in the hospital with ketoacidosis from high blood sugar. Why wasn't I? I don't know. What I do know, is that number stared me in the face despite consistent urine tests showing negative. I was in a swirl of confusion. Lindy and Dr. Guthrie explained to me that somehow my renal threshold had increased. Instead of filtering glucose out of my kidneys at the usual level, blood glucose around one hundred sixty to one hundred eighty, I wasn't "spilling" sugar until my blood glucose was higher...much, much higher.

I had had two back surgeries for my scoliosis in the months just prior to the A1c, and maybe my renal threshold changed due to the stress. Who knows? I'm still not sure what my renal threshold actually was, but I never did another urine test. Lindy got me a blood glucose meter to use until I could work with my insurance company to obtain payment for my own, and they may have saved my eyes, kidneys, and possibly even legs. The fear that coursed through me knowing that I had been doing everything "right", but was unknowingly going to hell in a hand-basket, emotionally reduced me to an amoeba. I have learned to depend on grace.

Today I wear a Glucowatch™ or use a small, simple accurate five second blood glucose tester that requires less blood than I lose squeezing a pimple. (Sorry...I was trying to make a point.) The Glucowatch™ is a small device worn on my arm (or ankle if I desire) that looks like a sports watch. It uses an electric current to measure interstitial fluid for glucose, and gives me a reading of my approximate blood glucose every ten minutes. Does it have drawbacks? Yes. Sometimes it is uncomfortable, irritates my skin or skips readings, and it requires two hours to calibrate to my skin before giving readings. How do I feel about wearing it or getting my blood sugar reading in five short seconds? I feel like I have come through the Dark Ages into the light. I can magically know what my blood sugar is in seconds. Harry Potter has no greater magic.

Well, back to the Biostator®. Using it was fascinating. It taught me how to think like a pancreas. The machine printed out blood sugar, and amount of insulin and/or glucose administered to the patient every minute.

People undergoing re-regulation came into the hospital the night before their twenty-four hour Biostator® run. The procedure was explained to them, and I devised an exercise plan and meal schedule to mimic their usual activity and food intake at home. They were hooked up to Bessie the Blue Biostator® (one of our pediatric patients felt she must have a name) at bedtime, and the games began.

The first few runs I stayed with the patient for twenty-four to thirty-six hours, because I wanted to see what the recordings said, as they came hot off the press. I was excited to learn how much insulin was required for individual patients doing specified exercise and eating specified amounts of food. The patients were interested as well. It was the perfect learning tool, because we got immediate personalized feedback.

Soon we learned that most patients needed increased insulin during the first ten to fifteen minutes of exercise, presumably due to release of stress hormones. Thereafter, the insulin requirement decreased, and Bessie gave glucose as the exercising muscle used sugar. Patients could see this happen on the recording right before their eyes. We also watched their blood glucose begin to rise as they ate, and Bessie pumped in the insulin. Within an hour or two after eating, Bessie fell back to administering minimal insulin or insulin as well as glucose.

These times between meals indicated basal (or baseline) insulin needs. The times Bessie pumped in lots of insulin during meals we called the bolus. At the end of twenty-four hours, Bessie's recording indicated the timing and amount of insulin the patient would need for a bolus of rapid acting insulin as well as baseline insulin. At home, baseline insulin would be provided by intermediate-acting insulin such as NPH® or Lente®, or a long-acting insulin such as Ultralente®. Ultralente® usually won out, as it had less peak action and longer duration, which translated into less fear of low blood sugar.

Mention of all these insulins seems weird these days, because of the explosion of new insulins that has nearly replaced them. In 2000, a new insulin called Lantus® became available that has no pronounced peak and lasts approximately twenty-four hours. Another basal insulin is Levemir®, which seems to have a bigger peak than Lantus®. Both are lovely options for basal insulin.

Bolus insulin for meals was provided by Regular insulin, which was the most rapid acting insulin available at the time. Now Apidra®, Humalog® or Novolog® are available as more rapid-acting insulins for the bolus. For your reference, Table 1 in the back of this book shows the most currently available insulins. Just remember that new ones may become available soon (maybe sooner than this book gets published!), and others are taken off the market. For example, Ultralente is currently unavailable in many markets, and soon will be an extinct species.

It was tremendously fun to show patients what their blood glucose had done over the twenty-four hour period, and explain how their basal and bolus insulins would mimic Bessie's administration for their home regimen.

Bessie usually administered about fifty percent more insulin than would be required in an injection regimen, because she was "chasing" the blood sugar. More insulin is required to lower an elevated blood glucose, than to prevent elevation and maintain normal blood glucose. At home however, patients would give their injections prior to meals, *preventing* blood glucose elevation.

Usually patients and their family members went home happy, and excited to implement a regimen they thought would work, because they actually saw the numbers, and Bessie had taught them how to think like a pancreas. Spending a full twenty-four hours with a patient and their family gave a lot of bonding time, too. We would swap stories about having diabetes, what a pain it was, and what we had learned from it. With the teenage kids it sometimes turned into a kind of Truth-or-Dare game. We would tell the dumbest things we had done with diabetes, and how we managed to come through it. Often there were misty eyes and tremendous appreciation for comradeship in a disease that required twenty-four/seven vigilance, and more rules to live by (lest you surely die) than Hoyles' Handbook. Let me be clear about whose eyes were misty: sometimes it was the patients' – *always* it was mine.

By the time these folks went home we were all fully invested in making a change for the better in how diabetes was treated: at a personal level and in the bigger picture, for all diabetic people everywhere. And I found new friends on this bizarre Diabetes Journey. In case any of you reading this book are people who endured twenty-four hours on the Biostator® with me, as the ever-present shadow to Bessie, let me tell you something...you inspired me. You encouraged me. You taught me. You were family.

Using the Biostator® for patients undergoing surgery was a bit more stressful than research or obstetric runs. It took an hour to boot up Bessie and get her running. Then the patient IVs were started and blood glucose had to be normalized before going into surgery. This usually took another hour or more. Our surgeries for diabetic patients started at six-thirty a.m. Are you getting the picture? My alarm clock went off at three a.m. on nights before surgery. It was intense.

Then there were the surgeons to deal with. Those of you who have spent a lot of time around Operating Rooms (OR's) know what I'm talking about. The surgeons I worked with were pretty high strung. Until they were used to working with the Biostator® in their OR, it was an Unknown, thus a threat. Since they did not feel comfortable barking at a machine in their favorite tones of irritation-covered-fear, they shared those with me. Sometimes quite loudly.

On the other hand, when the Biostator® kept their patient's blood sugar normalized during and after surgery, they became the big hero. Much was at stake as you can see, and often it was a definite love/hate relationship. Once they had seen the Biostator® work four or five times, they were glad to see Bessie and me coming. Then all I had to worry about was getting up at three a.m.

Using the Biostator® to control blood sugar for women going through Labor and Delivery (L & D) was wonderful. Shortly after starting the Biostator® program, our Pediatric Diabetes Team began a collaborative clinic with the Obstetricians for women who had diabetes during pregnancy. We, the diabetes people, were the Insulin Gurus, and the Obstetricians were the Pregnancy Wizards. Together we were a potent team.

Dr. Lois Jovanovic, of Sansum Research Foundation, in the 1980's, authored a cookbook type manual of appropriate diagnosis and care of diabetes for the pregnant woman. The cover of the book was deep eggplant purple, and The Purple Book served as our diabetes-and-pregnancy Bible. I have since heard people say that purple is a symbolic color for spirit or spiritual. I can tell you The Purple Book made that kind of difference for our pregnant diabetic moms and their babies.

To say that I enjoyed this clinic, and helping these mothers attain normal blood sugar throughout their pregnancy and delivery, would be like mentioning Niagara Falls as a dynamic little stream. I helped these women through education and coaching on insulin adjustment. Calling them or seeing them weekly in clinic, we always shared laughs, tears and/or encouragement. The fact that this helped bring about pink, healthy, normal weight, shrieking babies sometimes awed me to the core. In retrospect, those were powerful days: not powerful as in using force, but powerful in knowing within that I was a catalyst for good. And I wouldn't have done it, if I'd never gotten diabetes. Weird.

An additional benefit of Bessie and my presence in L & D was the calming effect it gave to the laboring moms, as well as the L & D staff. Everybody could relax (this is a relative term for the laboring mom) and do the work they were there to do, without worrying about the blood glucose either spiking or doing a crash-and-burn act. Not only that, I was a familiar advocate for the laboring mom, and Bessie and I stayed with her from start to finish. There were even a few babies named Rachel. Wow.

My years with the diabetes team were vastly educational - sometimes for our patients, *always* for me. I learned much about diabetes from a scientific perspective, and became more conscious of what was required for the spirit to thrive with this disease. Patients landed in our offices with courage, fear, fury, and sometimes hilarity. Parents often were tense, and their teenagers even more tense. These kids would ask me point-blank, in front of their parents, Dr. Brain, and whoever else might be in the exam room, what it *really* was like to have diabetes.

Yikes! The first time that happened I had to swallow hard and ask them to let me collect my thoughts. What I realized, was that I did not want to think about what it was *really* like to have diabetes. I had shoved that baggage in the deep freeze and replaced it with a zeal to *change* the way diabetes was treated. I was on a *Mission*! I had to save *all* of us! I wanted to be the diabetes *professional* who had it *all figured out* and the bad times were in the *past!* (I often thought in italics and exclamation marks during these times.)

So...here is what I thought. I hated this disease. I hated that it could kill me. I hated that it controlled so much of my schedule. I hated that I could not just be normal...whatever that was. I hated, that in many ways, it was such a dictator. And I hated the fact that despite all my vigilance...it still might steal about five years of my life, with the last ten years possibly being miserable. Heavy sigh.

On the other hand, it had taught me. I was more in tune with my body than most people. I could tell low blood sugar shakes and sweats from normal jitters or, as I mentioned before, just having the hots for a guy. I knew more about exercise and glucose metabolism than most people would in a lifetime. I knew it at a personal level. I was a runner. Okay, I was really a jogger. Actually I sort of jogged and walked... and I had done scientific research on it.

From an early age I had a Mission in life. A Guide. I wanted to help people with diabetes. I wanted to change the way diabetes was treated, especially from an emotional point of view. This guide that was with me always, reminded me of my Mission with every injection, test for sugar, meal plan, workout, annual doctor visit – day-in-and-day-out. I *knew* what I wanted to do. I shared this with the kids as we saw each other in clinic over the years. It helped us both.

I think back on my Deal with God. I know there are folks out there who think making a Deal with God is inadvisable, immoral or impossible. I think God leaves room for negotiation. My Deal was, "I will do everything I possibly can to keep myself as healthy as I can, if You will let me live long enough to know *why* You gave me this disease." We've both kept our bargains. I found my purpose, and I'm still alive. There were times I forgot God was keeping God's part of the deal. Or I forgot the deal altogether. Then something would come along: a new job, new opportunity, meaningful conversation with someone – and I would remember. We were both still on track.

Lessons Learned:
1. In my world, research laboratories are for...well, rats.
2. My lab inability is superseded, only by my mechanical incompetence.
3. It's true I slept with a dog, but don't tell anybody. That's just for you to know.
4. Bessie taught me how to think like a pancreas.
5. I agree with the ancient saying, "The teacher and the pupil are the lesson".

CHAPTER 22

One time when I thought I or maybe God had taken a detour, was when I began working with growth hormone research in our Pediatric Endocrinology clinic. This seemed totally irrelevant to diabetes. (Buzzzz! Wrong answer, but thank you for playing.)

Kids who have growth hormone deficiency are short. Remember the song about short people back in the 1980s? One phrase says, "...short people got no reason to live." Yes, it's a satire. Where does satire come from? Prejudices that really exist. So kids with short stature and people with diabetes have something in common—neither is normal...whatever that is.

Also, kids who need growth hormone have to take it by injection. Our research protocol included either daily injections or injections three times weekly. As I taught moms of these kids how to inject their children, the fear in their eyes was the same as the fear I saw in the moms of diabetic children. I remember one incident with a boy I will call Opie.

Opie was very short for his age. His shortness stuck out like a sore thumb when you realized how old he was. The thing is, most people did not realize how old he was, even after they knew. They mistook him for being younger, and treated him that age. When I met Opie he was eleven years old, but had the size and physical maturation of a six year old. Are you imagining how he was treated?

Not only adults treated him like he was six; his classmates did, too. Some of them bullied him incessantly, others treated him like the class mascot and carried him around on their shoulders. Either way, Opie was not normal. Cute? Indubitably. Normal? Not on your life.

When Opie and his mom came to clinic I could see her strain. Opie's tension did not register as openly as his mom's. Maybe he learned to hide it better, since he had to deal with it every minute of every day. I began to talk about growth hormone, and how it might help Opie's growth catch up with other kids his age, within a few years. Opie became noticeably more interested; his mom smiled and dabbed at her eyes. They wanted to try it.

Then came giving the first injection. Opie was a fairly easy-going boy, and his mom a practical, down-to-earth woman. We reconstituted the vial of growth hormone and drew it into the syringe. She had practiced once on an orange, and now it was time for a target much softer, and nearer and dearer to her heart. I explained that the faster the needle went through the skin the less "discomfort" it would cause.

"Discomfort" is a word we often use in the health care profession to make ourselves believe we do not cause people pain. The patients however, know the difference. Regardless, Opie's mom very quickly plunged the needle into his arm, and despite her practical nature, nearly fainted. Opie looked on, astonished.

"Mom! I didn't even feel that! Really, I'm not kidding. Wow!"

Tears escaped and fled down Opie's mom's cheeks. She injected the growth hormone and removed the needle.

"Mom, I'm not kidding. That didn't hurt!" Opie was clearly ecstatic.

His mom slumped into the nearest chair and wiped the tears from her chin.

This was the same reaction our diabetic kids and their parents had. Syringes and needles had improved drastically since I was a kid. Needles were tiny in diameter and siliconized, so they literally slid through the skin. It was almost as easy as brushing your teeth. But oh, the *look*, the *thought* of a needle! It strikes the same effect as a poisonous viper of immense proportions. It courses terror through the veins of the most stalwart, and all present know this shot situation is *not* normal.

I started to realize there's no such thing as normal. Short stature, diabetes, you name it; we all have something outside of normal. Let me tell you what Webster's says about *normal*. First of all, there are five (count them...1-2-3-4-5) different definitions. And quite frankly none of them sound alike. If normal was so ubiquitous, wouldn't there be only one definition?

The first definition, to which we as a culture desperately subscribe, is to "conform to an accepted standard, model or pattern, especially one corresponding to the median or average of a large group". *WHAT??!!* All that says is that we take a bunch of people, smoosh them into a wad, and lop off anything that sticks out as not-normal. Then we define the smooshed wad as the standard everyone is supposed to *conform to*. It's a *joke*. Normal only exists in numbers, it is not something a person can BE.

All things considered, I think I would rather be an out-lier, thank you very much. I enjoy the idea of *conforming to* someone else's idea of normal almost as much as I enjoy the thought of *compliance*, and we've already discussed that. As you can see, I'm getting wound up; it's what we thinkers do.

Have you ever heard healthcare people talk about a "compliant" or "noncompliant" diabetic? Often they forget that diabetic is an adjective, not a noun, and definitely not a *person*. In listening to such an oration, one might assume that a compliant diabetic most surely will go to heaven and live happily ever after. They are the ones who do what the healthcare people tell them to without questioning, and come back to clinic with stellar results such as weight loss, a normal fasting blood sugar and fresh clean breath. (Okay, I threw in the breath part to emphasize a point.) Well, excuse me, but what about the folks who do what they are told and it does not work? Huh? Then we have to actually *think*, which is oh-so-noncompliant. This discussion reminds me of Jennie, my hospital roommate. She was wise beyond her years.

The second definition of normal has to do with "occurring naturally". Well, now there's an issue. What exactly, is "naturally"? I would say diabetes happened to me pretty naturally. I did not buy it. I did not go looking for it. It just came. Poof! So, by that definition, I see an argument for saying diabetes *is* normal. The same is true for short stature. It just happens. For some kids you can trace back to a causative factor, but then the argument ensues that the causative factor might have been natural for them as well. Who can say?

The third definition has to do with hydrogens, salts, and acids, and the fourth definition has to do with being perpendicular. These come from the fields of chemistry and math consecutively. They do not seem to apply to our current discussion, so I wish them well.

However, the fifth definition seems to spin a never-ending spiral. It comes from the fields of medicine and psychology and states, "...free from disease, disorder, or malformation; sound." Okay, stay with me for a moment here. According to this definition, if I get a cold I am no longer normal. If my house is a disorderly mess, I am no longer normal. If the thumbnails on my right and left hands do not match I am not normal. Which they don't, but that is beside the point, because the fact that I've had colds, a disorderly house and diabetes, kicked me out of normal long ago.

Am I the only one who thinks there is something exceptionally arbitrary about this definition? If it is so arbitrary, then why should I care if I fit or not? I was born and raised a people-pleaser, so such thinking has taken much time and turmoil to surface. Yet (and this is a big YET...) I wonder if it leads down the road to freedom. And if it does, diabetes started my wondering, so...

... maybe having diabetes is leading me to freedom.

Lessons Learned:

1. Is short stature as hard to deal with as diabetes? It probably depends on which you have.
2. The look of a shot may be far worse than the feel of a shot, but it is hard to separate the two when you're terrified.
3. Normal is a trumped up definition that is not applicable to living breathing Beings.

CHAPTER 23

I was feeling pretty comfortable managing diabetes for both my patients and myself, when diabetes struck, yet again. The doctor told Mom she had a "little sugar." A little sugar? Isn't that like being a little pregnant?

"Mom, what does that mean? What's he saying?"

"Well, he says not to worry, it's not very high right now."

"How high is 'not very high'?"

"Oh, he said just about two hundred or so."

"Two hundred?! Mom, that's high."

"Kind of high, but Dr. Meanswell said he wouldn't put 'diabetes' on my chart, because then I'd have trouble with the insurance company. He doesn't want to put me on medication yet."

I was going nowhere, but getting there fast. By this time, Janis had completed two degrees, one of which was in nursing, and despite both our concerns Mom went without treatment for several years. With two nurses in the family, Dad and Holly stayed out of the soap opera, leaving action items to us. Hemoglobin A1c testing was still new, and not widely utilized, especially in the general practice arena, so none of us really knew what Mom's blood sugars were. When she finally got an A1c, after adamantly demanding it from her physician (Mom was scary when she got riled), it was ten percent. Oh my.

Mom having diabetes seemed impossible, yet natural. Impossible, because according to the research back then, the tendency for type 1 and type 2 diabetes are carried on different genes. It was unusual to have both types in one family. That's when I began to wonder a lot about how much more we do NOT know about diabetes, than what we do. How much of what we believe about health is actually as archaic as bleeding people?

Mom having diabetes completed the circle of diabetic women in our immediate family. We were all in the same boat. Mom had spent most of her adult life dealing with diabetes, and hoping for a cure for her children.

Can your mind be on something so fervently without it affecting your body? Things that make you go "Hmm."

Mom asked her doctor to start oral medication, which he *finally* did. Did I mention "*finally*"? During this time Dad's heart attacks were increasing in frequency, so Mom's attention was diverted to his health; the age-old story of being a woman. Several years later when she came up for air and got another A1c, it was around eleven percent. This got all of us motivated. Mom needed insulin.

One would think that any physician staring at an A1c of eleven percent in a patient, who had diabetes for several years, would immediately consider insulin. One would be wrong. At least back in the 1990s. Sadly enough, it still happens today, but thankfully, less often.

Janis and I gave Mom our best pep talks, to convey to her physician, but they went over like a dead balloon. Then Janis called him. Then I called him. Then I sent him a three inch binder filled with articles from professional peer-reviewed diabetes journals discussing A1c and the need for insulin in someone with type 2 diabetes. Finally, we got Mom on insulin, and her A1c went down to slightly less than seven percent, although she still had to demand that he order the tests. Please.

I learned a lot from Mom's diabetes. I had been living in a little bubble within the subspecialty of Pediatric Endocrinology within a huge academic tertiary care center. A place where people go to find the specialists' specialist. I thought everybody got treatment and education for diabetes that included the latest standards of care. I was wrong.

Another thing I learned is, *Do not give diabetic advice to your Mom.* It uselessly expends energy. One day Mom called me.

"Hi Sweetie! I'm having trouble with my blood sugars, can you help me out?"

This is every good-daughter's dream, to have your Mom actually ask you for help in an area that is your specialty. She told me what was happening with her blood sugars, when they were going high and low, and the problem was predictable. It was one I treated several times daily for our patients. I gave her my sage advice.

There was dead air on the phone.

Then Mom said, (and I quote) "Oh. Thanks honey, but I'm sure that's not right."

I have learned to turf her to Janis.

Mom had trouble identifying when she had low blood sugar. This was a scary thing, because she sometimes got too low, and became confused, forgetting how to treat herself. One day Mom called.

"Hi Mom!"

"Rachel, I'm feeling really low today." This came in a very subdued and quiet voice.

I panicked, but fought it off bravely by overwhelming myself with logic. "Mom, where are you?"

"In the kitchen."

"Good! Okay Mom, walk to the refrigerator. Can you hear me?"

"Um...yes."

"Okay, open the door. Do you have any juice?"

"No."

"That's okay. Do you have milk?"

"Yes."

"Okay Mom. Take a big drink of milk right out of the carton. Its okay, you don't need a glass, just take a big slug of milk. Are you doing that?"

(...glug) "Yes."

"Great! Just keep drinking Mom, you're doing great." At this point if she passed out, at least she would have something in her gut to eventually raise her blood sugar. I could hear her dutifully slurping the milk. "Okay Mom, take the carton with you and sit down. Can you do that?"

"Yes, there's a chair here."

"Good. Do you feel dizzy?"

"No."

"That's good." My panic was slowly receding; but just in case, I made back up plans. If she trailed off mid-sentence I'd call 911, give them her address and tell them her status. "How are you feeling Mom? Is your head clearing?"

"My head's fine, Rachel. Nothing's wrong with my head."

"Oh. Were you just feeling weak and couldn't think right?"

"No."

"No? How did you know to call me?"

"Sweetie, I'm just feeling really *low* because I got word today my friend Jacqueline passed away. I needed to talk to somebody."

I'm sure Jacqueline was pleased to look down from heaven and see the hysterical laughter she provided for Mom and me.

Lessons Learned:

    1.   Why did Mom have to get diabetes too? You tell me, and we'll both know.

    2.   Living with diabetes brings new interpretations to the English language.

CHAPTER 24

After twelve years at KUMC, I began to feel that nudge of impatience again; it was time to do the next thing. I had significant experience doing clinical research with new pharmaceutical compounds (growth hormone and insulin), so I checked out opportunities at a Kansas City based pharmaceutical company, Marion Merrell Dow (MMD). I also checked out a company in San Francisco called Genentech. Moving to San Francisco sounded both exciting and scary. Leaving my friends was the scariest part.

The past few years had bestowed an additional upheaval in my life. The man, who in college had convinced me marriage was a good idea, now had slowly, persistently and irrevocably convinced me it was not. He moved on, and I was foot-loose and fancy-free, so why not go for the Big Move?

In my heart the local company felt better.

I applied for the local position in clinical research, and went through several rounds of interviews, which I felt went well. After several weeks and more phone interviews I was sure I had the job!

Shortly thereafter the company instituted a hiring freeze.

Three months later, their freeze thawed, and interviews started all over again. I got a little ragged. Finally, after six months I got a letter from MMD (I was now on nickname basis). I laid the unopened letter on the counter and contemplated it over a strong cup of coffee. If I was hired, life had new direction, excitement, more travel (which at that time I considered positively), new people, new friends, new faces, being part of Corporate America! If I was not hired...hmm. Maybe better to have dinner first and read the letter on a full stomach.

But *surely* I was offered a position! Something inside me said MMD was my Next Place. They were starting research with a new compound for diabetes, and hardly anyone in the company had diabetes experience. Voila! Here I am with enough diabetes experience to bedazzle the masses – what better choice could exist?

After dinner and a few more hours of dialogue inside my Brain-of-Many-Voices, I carefully opened what I decided was the Letter of Acceptance. I was wrong. I was devastated.

My newly formed Brain Trust told me all the reasons I should *not* be devastated. This made me not only more devastated, but guilt-laden for being devastated, and mad that I had to pretend I was not.

Fine! Apparently this was God's will (a phrase often used when devastating things happen). Apparently I should stay at KUMC...but my gut, now joining the cacophony of the Brain Trust, yelled "Wrong!" Yet nobody knew where I *should* go.

Night fell - morning came, and I marched off to work at the Medical Center again, still in a quandary. A few days passed and another letter in an MMD envelope arrived. What is this? They feared I did not understand the first brush off, so they sent a follow up? I ripped open the following letter:

Dear Ms. Gifford:

I am pleased to inform you that we would like you to join our research team at Marion Merrell Dow. Please contact our Health office at the number below for a complete entry physical and drug screen at your earliest convenience.

Blah, blah, etc.

Sincerely,

Ms. Somebody

Queen of Human Resources

What?! Apparently I was not the only one with a Schizophrenic Brain Trust. I called the number in a semi-hostile mood. If there was anything I disliked more than being jerked around, it was to go to the doctor, especially an unknown doctor, and they had the nerve to include both in less than a full paragraph.

"Hello, this is Rachel Gifford, and I just received a letter asking me to schedule a physical exam as the final step before working at MMD. I am confused." Confused was the word I chose over a less socially acceptable one. There was silence for a moment, during which time I probably should have been considering how to soften my approach, but instead was gathering mental ammunition for onslaught.

"Ms. Gifford, Mr. McDermott would like for you to join his research team."

I remembered Stan McDermott. I had thoroughly enjoyed speaking with him in our interview. But what was this crap about a physical? Like I didn't see the doctor enough as it was? Hmff.

"Let me clarify something with you." I considered perhaps Ms. Somebody did not know the whole story. "Less than a week ago I received a letter stating I would not be joining MMD. This came after six months of interviewing with the company in person and via phone, a hiring freeze, more interviews (I gave her the roller coaster saga)...and *now* I receive a letter abruptly telling me to schedule a physical with someone who is not my own personal physician as part of my entry to the company. *What*, exactly is this all about?"

Silence. "Uh, Ms. Gifford, you seem upset."

Upset did not even start to cover it. "I am quite upset. I have been interested in working with your company, but I am not in the least interested in being jerked around." There, I said it. Quick body-check for remorse: none apparent.

Interestingly enough Ms. Somebody did not hang up on me, and ultimately we came to the clarification that I had indeed been denied a position by one team, but Stan McDermott's team wanted me. His was the team heading up the diabetes compound. Happy days, oh happy days! I signed up.

I mired through this long and circuitous story for a reason. It is more and more apparent to me that diabetes is a major "tool" I got, to help me learn the lessons I have for this life. Everybody gets one or two. Although Gut told me I was headed to MMD, the data gave me a different story, causing my Brain Trust significant turmoil (Read: Agony). What was Real however, never changed.

At MMD I got quarterly reviews with annual pay raises, profit sharing and bonus packages. We all had a personal computer on our desktops (this was 1991, so that was not the norm it is today), and whenever I needed educational books I was told to "just order it". Any of you who have worked in a government institution will understand my astonishment.

There was no personal or professional inquisition; there was no questioning of *why* I needed this textbook nor a twenty-five page form to complete promising my soul in return. For some reason, they just trusted my word. Really.

Doing clinical research in such a place made me certain I had died and gone to heaven. I collaborated with nationally and internationally recognized diabetes researchers. The authors I read in diabetes journals were now real people I knew on a first name basis. I helped them set up studies and periodically visited to review their data and give them study updates. Getting to know these physicians and their diabetes team members was beyond thrilling. Several became wonderful friends, and I totally enjoyed this diabetes kindredship.

After two years of living in Nirvana, corporate reorganization reared its ugly head. What I know now that I did not know then, is that reorganization and regurgitation have similar meanings. In both situations something that has a comfortable spot in life, knows its path, and is peacefully headed there, is interrupted, intercepted and interjected into a new location...sometimes landing in the dumper.

After the reorganization we were R.I.F.'ed, which stood for Reduction in Force, unless you can imagine some of the other creative things we decided it meant. The "F" on the end was great fertilizer for creating meaningful phrases.

A few months later we were R.I.F.'ed again, and the rumor besieged like wildfire that we were "slimming down for the wedding"; the company was planning to merge. As with most rumors, there is always a grain of truth. In our case the grain was the size of Germany, and our new company became a merger of Hoechst Roussel and Marion Merrell Dow, dubbed Hoechst Marion Roussel. Absolutely no one in the United States could correctly pronounce Hoechst unless they had studied several years of German, so we quickly became HMR in conversational discussions...of which there were many.

During this time, I felt that nudge again. It was not all that gentle this time, as I had shoved squarely up against a glass ceiling that was crushing my brain. I needed something new, whether it was a different company or different department within the same company. I needed a less patriarchally dominated arena or I was going to explode.

Health Outcomes Research was becoming a very hot topic in the pharmaceutical industry, and our company was in the thick of it. As a generality, Health Outcomes Research (HOR for short...not a good acronym) uses several methods of collecting and analyzing data regarding the cost of patient care, versus the outcomes a patient receives from that care. Then a quantified cost analysis could be done. The HOR fervor was fueled by the rising cost of healthcare, and the government's tendency to point their finger at pharmaceutical companies as the ultimate culprit, despite the fact the Pentagon was buying five-thousand dollar hammers. HMR had started a new Health Outcomes Research department, and was looking for people with research experience. I applied.

This was another time when things moved very slowly. The company was still reeling from their last merger, so transfer positions were on hold. After four months that seemed like an eternity, I started doing Health Outcomes studies in diabetes. Initially I worked on compounds that were not yet approved by the FDA, collecting and analyzing data to help in cost-effective pricing, once approval was obtained. The work was a little slow, so I kept my eyes open for opportunities.

HOR suddenly got a new Director. It is an odd story, but a woman joined the department as a PhD intern, and within a few weeks jumped three promotions and became Director. As you might guess some people in our department were puzzled, while others over whom she had leap-frogged, bordered on hysteria. Being new to the department, I decided to keep my head down and go with the flow.

As the flow would have it, our new Director began building the group, and I saw an opportunity to go from working with drugs prior to FDA approval, to drugs that had already been approved. In essence this would take me from "research" to "marketing", a quantum leap in mindset. For example: research is interested in data and drug approval, research people pinch pennies until they scream, and research people are often a rather quiet lot. Although I never fit the quiet mode, the rest agreed with my upbringing.

Marketing is on the other end of the spectrum. Their motto is, "You have to spend money to make money". The more you spend the more you make, and marketing people are *LOUD* and *RAMBUNCTIOUS* and *Movers 'n Shakers!* Despite some trepidation, I took the new position.

Immediately I traveled more. I met with physicians across the nation who wanted funding for outcomes studies. I funded them, and designed the studies. I was Movin' 'n Shakin' fer sher...and having a great time! I also learned that people in marketing often have a higher income than people in research. Not a bad thing.

I Moved 'n Shook for a few months, and then our company decided to relaunch a diabetes drug. The drug originally launched during the most recent merger, and consequently fell through the cracks. A large part of the problem occurred because the drug was our first move into the diabetes market place. Our sales and marketing people did not know the national diabetes thought-leaders' names, let alone have a relationship with them.

They targeted marketing to primary care physicians first, instead of endocrinologists who were diabetes specialists. In a way this makes sense, as primary care doctors see the largest number of diabetic patients. However, bypassing the specialists in diabetes, was...um...not well received. (Read: Fried them to a crisp.)

During this time I met with the Marketing Director of diabetes, to offer my services via Outcomes research. I let her know of my relationships with many of the diabetes thought-leaders from prior years in diabetes research, and that I would be happy to help in any way I could.

Her response was unexpected, "Why don't you become the Professional Education Manager for diabetes?"

I had a clever response. "Uh...no, that's not...er...what does that job really mean?"

She called my HOR Director the next day and discussed the transfer opportunity. That afternoon the Professional Education Director called me and requested a meeting. Without further ado, I was invited to become Professional Education Manager for diabetes. Holy cow! Is this how things move in marketing?

My mind went from zero to sixty in about two nanoseconds. I learned the Professional Education Manager was in charge of working with the national healthcare key opinion leaders, or KOL's as they're anacronymically called. Managers support healthcare professional education, and do other educational stuff; stuff being a technical term for all those things I did not yet know. It meant fifty to sixty percent travel, and I had just started a doctorate program. How would that work?

Here's how our interview went:

Pro Ed Director (smiling pleasantly in an outgoing sales-person sort of way): "Do you have experience organizing scientific meetings and educational symposia?"

Me: "A little."

Director: "I understand you are familiar with most of the national diabetes thought-leaders?"

Me: "Yes, I've worked with them for several years."

Director: "Do you enjoy meeting and talking science with diabetes physicians?"

Me: "Um...yes, it's terrific."

Director: "Well, then this is exactly the position for you!"

Me: (looking around the room, to see who she addressed) "Um... well..."

Smooth words like, *Let me get back to you* or *I need some time to fully consider this opportunity* escaped me. What I knew of the position sounded interesting and terrifying. I decided to act like a marketing person: I pushed for more money.

Lessons Learned:

1. Where I am supposed to be, I will end up.
2. Sometimes Brain Trust is a liar, whereas Gut knows the bigger Truth. Does God speak Gut?
3. Leaping from research to marketing crosses several boundaries, and feels similar to moving from the bayou to downtown Manhattan.

CHAPTER 25

A small fact no one had shared with me prior to entering the position of Manager of Diabetes Professional Education, was the *extent* to which endocrinologists were angry with our company. I spent the first six months of my new job listening to endocrinologists tell me we were idiots, and they would never work with us in any way. Those were the nice things they said.

I responded by listening quietly, letting them know I knew we had made a mistake, but that I knew we could change it. How could they help me turn things around? After a few months, the tide began to turn. Because I had long-time friendships with many of these physicians, they believed me, and indeed, they began to help us. I was grateful, and shortly thereafter able to discontinue my ulcer medication.

That year, 1997, I traveled fifty percent of weekdays, as well as being gone fifty percent of weekends. When in the office, most days lasted twelve to fourteen hours, trying to catch up.

I also remarried that year. Randy and I married on July second, took the long holiday weekend, and I was back in the office Monday morning bright and early. My doctoral program became a casualty, and on occasion I remembered at one time I had been a sane person with a life.

The job was the best of times and the worst of times.

Worst: Relentless travel.

Best: Traveled to beautiful places, and mixed business with pleasurable surroundings.

Worst: Often I saw only the *inside* of hotel and meeting rooms in the beautiful places.

Worst: Initially, endocrinologists were furious with HMR, and I was the designated ear of the company.

Best: Once they softened, working with them was delightful.

Best: The challenge of resurrecting a sinking ship brought more personal satisfaction than simply hailing a seaworthy vessel.

Worst: Work hours were ridiculous.

Best: I could talk diabetes science with these brilliant people for hours on end.

Long after meetings were over, and into the night, we would talk, over drinks and fine cigars (I always had a cigar...sometimes they did, too), discussing probable, possible and sometimes magical things in the world of diabetes. It was a natural high. These people were Thinkers; I had found home turf.

On one of these late-night-science-discussion-evenings, Dr. Julio Rosenstock, who is one of the loveliest characters (and I do mean *character*) I am happy to call my friend, waved his cigar at me and leaned forward. In his thick Costa Rican accent, he said, "Rrrachel...about this diabetes drug HMR launched: the firrrst time, you deedn't rrreally *launch* your drug. You just sort of poooshed it off the end of the pier!" Well said, Julio...well said.

I spent five high energy years loving my job as Professional Education Manager for diabetes. During these years, having diabetes was more of an asset than a liability. What a role-reversal! In 1999 the company merged, yet again, to become Aventis, and made the decision to move from Kansas City to New Jersey. Because of the company's history in Kansas City, a great sadness coursed through all of us.

Marion Laboratories, the original Kansas City company of Marion Merrell Dow, was started by Ewing Marion Kauffman, a daring and uncommon entrepreneur. He began his pharmaceutical business in the 1950s, crushing up oyster shells in his basement by night, and selling Oscal® by day, long before FDA stringencies became what they are now. He borrowed one thousand dollars from five of his friends for capital. When he sold the company these men became multi-millionaires. Mr. "K", as he was lovingly called, believed that "those who shared in the work should share in the rewards". He set up a stock option program providing shares for everyone from the CEO to the janitorial staff. Maintenance workers loved to tell how they sent their children to college on Mr. K's stocks.

The company was like a huge family, run by a benevolent and exceptionally wealthy father of fine principles. Mr. K bought the Kansas

City Royals, because he felt a city must have a professional baseball team to be "on the map" for business. His Marion family benefited from the Royals purchase, because every year he hosted Marion-Night-at-the-Royals. An entire section was reserved for Marion associates (we were not employees - worker bees of the world - we were all equivalent associates providing a crucial element to the business), and everything was free, from parking and entry tickets, all the way down to the last hot dog and bag of popcorn! It was the greatest family reunion you could imagine.

Mr. Kauffman had another phenomenal annual event called *Marion on the Move.* Each year on the celebration day, buses would line up in front of our office buildings, and transport every employee downtown to the Convention Center. We all got a box lunch, and sat listening to live, high-energy music, from famous bands of the time, waiting for Mr. K. to come to the stage. Before he entered, a hush fell over the room, and excitement was palpable.

In he came! Music blared, tingles ran down your spine, hair stood on end. When Mr. K spoke about the Marion Family, you knew you were the Best-of-the-Best, the Proud, the True, the Brave. He called his company an Uncommon Company, built on Uncommon principles, and it was. To watch this culture end, and move from Kansas City was crushing. Yet inevitable.

About seven percent of the company moved to New Jersey. Initially Randy and I planned to be part of the Exodus. I had friends in the east and it would have been an exciting adventure. However, the more we looked into it, the more difficult the picture became. Each day Randy would have to drive an hour or more toward Newark for work; I would drive an hour or more in the opposite direction for work. We would add more than two hours to each workday, which already was long. Housing prices were about fifty percent higher in New Jersey, and salaries were not being compensated to cover the inflationary increase. And then, that little nudge came again.

This time it was not impatience. It was more of an impression inside my heart that drifted up to my head, saying, *It's time to do your own thing.* There are those who would consider starting a company way too scary.

Had I thought more about it, I would have been one of those. For the first time in my life, I did not think. I listened.

My Professional Education position transitioned to New Jersey in July 2000. I stayed in Kansas City, and incorporated DM Strategies in August. DM stands for Diabetes Mellitus. I labored over our company Mission Statement, trying to say something personally meaningful, novel, yet corporate sounding. All I knew was, I wanted to change the way diabetes is treated.

When I say "change", I mean in several ways. From a psychological viewpoint, I want to change how the *people* with the disease are treated. It is not uncommon for people with type 2 diabetes to be covertly (sometimes overtly) blamed for having the disease. Our culture in general, and healthcare professionals as well, see an overweight person with type 2 diabetes, and tend to lay fault, guilt, and blame on the patient. Stuffing a patient with guilt is like over-packing a gun with black powder; sooner or later it's gonna go off, and neither the gun nor the stuffer will benefit.

I wanted patients to get the initial and ongoing lifetime education they need to *really* know how to care for themselves with this disease. I wanted people to know their health belongs to them, seeing health care providers as their coaches and encouragers.

This was a huge challenge, because our current health care system is not set up that way. It is formatted to deal with short-term illnesses that get better and go away after a few pills, shots or IVs. The healthcare system is the do-er, seeing the patient as the do-ee. That does not work for a disease where the do-ee is, in fact, the do-er of the disease twenty-four hours every day, seven days every week, day in and day out, no time off for vacation, holidays or good behavior. The current health care paradigm does not fit, and those of us with diabetes know it all too well.

I wanted to change how diabetes is treated from a therapeutic viewpoint, as well. Currently, we have a better armamentarium of diabetes therapies than has ever been available, but many physicians do not yet know how to sequence, dose or combine the drugs, nor how to monitor drug effectiveness. Most people with type 2 diabetes are cared for by primary care physicians, whose practices are so busy, it is impossible for the physician to know the latest therapeutic measures, let alone focus on all the needs of each diabetic patient, in the six to nine minutes allotted for patient visits. And they're still scared to start insulin. Oh my.

The worst part of this is they don't *know* they don't know, so they are not looking for answers. Instead, patients may receive the blame as being "noncompliant" (that nasty word again).

The United Kingdom Prospective Diabetes Study (UKPDS) studied people with newly diagnosed diabetes through ten years of their disease. It ended in 1997, and provided a vast amount of information about how these people are best treated. Studies are still being published as the data continue to be analyzed. One of the important realities the study discovered was that type 2 diabetic people ultimately will require insulin as part of their treatment for normalizing blood sugar, but physicians sometimes use insulin like a cattle prod.

In fact, I have actually seen a physician hold a syringe in-hand; shake it at his patient, and say, "If you don't do what I'm telling you to do with your diet and weight loss, I'm going to put you on *The Needle*."

I nearly threw up. Patients should not be threatened: period. People should not be threatened *especially*, with the very air they need to breathe.

Our ability to care for diabetes is greater than our ability to get information to the masses of physicians caring for diabetic people, and we are not even scratching the surface of educating the people themselves. This brings me to deep-seated feelings: I feel like crying, shrieking the frustration I feel for all of us who have this disease. And I feel a burning within to get the word out to our nation that is experiencing an increase in diabetes diagnoses at epidemic proportions. Get this: the Centers for Disease Control (CDC) predict that of people born in or after the year 2000, one in every three will develop diabetes in their life time. Does that stop you in your tracks?

All this boils down to the Mission Statement of my company: **Changing the way diabetes is treated** – at the national level – through education, research, public speaking and publication.

For years I have wanted to write a book about having diabetes, and learning to live with it. I wanted to write about making an alliance with

195

it, and realizing it was a tool I received in my life for helping me dig deep to find out who I was, and why I got dropped on this planet. I wanted to call it *Learning How to Think Like a Pancreas*. I thought that was pretty clever. I was wrong. When I told friends the title they gave me a blank stare, and changed the subject.

Okay, maybe it didn't' work for everybody.

Within a few weeks of incorporating DM Strategies I began to write this book. It was not in the original business plan; I considered it a hobby. The Real Work was educating health care professionals, to change the way diabetes is treated. The Real Work moved along, but the gentle urging to write this book got...well...less gentle. Ever been coerced off the road by an oncoming tractor trailer? It was that kind of gentle.

But wow...writing about myself was way more difficult than I thought it would be. Being honest about myself was hard. Sometimes simply uncovering my own truth was even harder. I have considered moving on to fiction.

Lessons Learned:
1. Fine cigars and science talk are excellent bonding tools.
2. It was sad to lose an Uncommon Company.
3. If you ever decide to write a book about yourself, have a lovely glass of wine, and lay down until the feeling goes away.

"The difficult I can do today. The impossible will take a little longer."
Billie Holiday, lady who sang the blues

Epilogue

I've heard it said that life is ten percent what you make it, and ninety percent how you take it. For me that has been oh-so-true. Diabetes hit me so hard, I've spent most of my life trying to make it an easier disease for other folks than it was for me. In high school Chemistry class I learned about catalysts, which basically are agents of change. I decided that's what I would be. In 2004, DM Strategies, Inc. was doing quite well, so I decided to take my next head-long leap, and started a nonprofit organization called Diabetes Freedom Foundation (DFF). I'll put some information about DM Strategies, Inc. and DFF at the end of this chapter.

You may be wondering about the name, with the words *Diabetes* and *Freedom* sitting right next to each other as oxymoronishly as *Artificial* and *Intelligence* sometimes do. Isn't that just another way to say Natural Stupidity? Perhaps. The point of DFF however, is ***freeing people from the tyranny of diabetes***. This could happen by gaining Freedom either *from* diabetes, *with* diabetes or *through* diabetes.

Most of what you have already read in this book talks about how I discovered freedom with, and through diabetes, so let's talk about freedom *from* diabetes, as that's a favorite topic of mine these days. How long do you think diabetes has been around? The precise answer is...a long, long time. It was first documented in Egyptian papyrus papers. Good grief. That says to me it is absolutely time for it to be gone. It's over-stayed its welcome. I feel in my gut the cure, the stoppage of this disease, is jumping up and down from behind the rock where it's been hiding, shrieking, *Here I am! Find me! Hide and seek is over!*

Research changes the world very slowly. You may have noticed that. But after a while a critical mass builds, and it's like a huge snowball rolling down hill – it gains speed like a freight train. I know I'm mixing metaphors, but you get the idea. As far back as 1988, a physician named Jesse Roth showed that insulin was being made in a one-celled laboratory animal specimen that **had no pancreas.** What?! That's what the scientific world said, too. They didn't believe him, and accused him of sloppy laboratory technique, such as not washing his test tubes well enough. It took years before they would even publish his information in research journals. After several other laboratories across the United States showed the same thing, they finally published his work. That is a pretty remarkable finding, and it points to the fact that insulin is made in many cells other than just the pancreas. Scientists today are pondering if it may be made in every cell of the body.

To further shake up the world of diabetes experts, in June 2005, research was reported at the annual American Diabetes Association (ADA) meeting showing that people who had lived with type 1 diabetes even as long as sixty years, were still making islet cells (the ones in the pancreas that make insulin). We've seen the slower rolling part of the snowball, but things are speeding up. Just one year later, 2006, researchers discovered that capsaicin, a derivative of hot chili peppers, cured diabetes in mice.

I love the story about how they discovered this. They had made some mice diabetic, and were studying the diabetic neuropathy the mice were developing, with hopes to heal the neuropathy. The researchers felt there might be an immunologic origin for the neuropathy, so they gave the mice capsaicin, as it had previously shown to reduce immune diseases. The next morning they came back to check the mice, and none of them had diabetes anymore! If you want to read more about this, the reference is Dosch, M. Cell, Vol 127, 1123-1135. The finding definitely points to diabetes having both immune and neurological origins, as well as endocrine origins. The experts in immune medicine, neurology and endocrinology are in disagreement about what is occurring, which is not a big surprise. Honestly, it's like disagreements among various religions on how to get to heaven.

However, another finding that points in the same direction was reported at the ADA in 2005. Researchers tried to get islet cells to replicate in a Petri dish. Keep in mind that islet cells are believed to be endocrine cells. The researchers had trouble getting them to replicate, but finally several of the bolder ones made babies, so to speak, despite the lack of privacy in a Petri dish. When the researchers looked at the new cells however, what they found were mostly....neurons! So, islet cells had baby nerve cells, as well as a few baby islet cells. Nerve cells and endocrine cells are siblings. That pretty much clenches the fact that diabetes is a neuro-immuno-endocrine disease.

That brings me to a very shocking thought. We know that different thoughts and emotions cause neurons to secrete different neurotransmitters, that go to the immune system with their messages of happiness, anger, fear, etc, and affect our immunity in helpful or not so helpful ways. What if my feelings can ultimately influence my immune system to no longer recognize my islet cells as being part of me, and thus attack them? Or perhaps cause islet cells to make more message-senders (neurons) than hormone secretors (islet cells).

It has long been documented that people developed type 1 diabetes after a great shock, loss or illness, substantiating an emotional impulse. A theory presented at the 2005 ADA by T.J. Wilkin, discussed type 1 and type 2 diabetes as the same disease, type 1 just happened faster. He called it the Acceleration Theory. So perhaps both type 1 and type 2 are immunologic. Makes sense to me.

After reading and noticing all these things, I truly wonder if there is a *personal* cure for diabetes. My childhood conclusion from watching my mom and sister was that the kid with the disease got the Mom. There is a certain irony in the fact that diabetes was actually my twelfth birthday present. On the day of my last pre-pubertal birthday, did I make a subconscious decision to make a final stab at getting the mom? Darned if I know, but to overlook that fact as irrelevant is like overlooking the fact that plants grow better when they get fertilizer.

There is far more to healing than medical intervention. The body and mind work together to heal. We know that patients with cancer improve more quickly if they do meditation and visual imaging of their cancer cells dying, and their bodies growing strong and healthy. *Kitchen Table Wisdom* written by Rachel Naomi Remen, MD, is an entire book dedicated to reporting such episodes of self-healing. Dr. Mitch Krucoff, a cardiologist at Duke University Medical Center, along with his associates, showed that heart patients who have people praying for them have shorter stays in the ICU and 25% to 30% better chance of survival than do those who do not receive prayer on their behalf. If you'd like to read more about his study, it can be found in the American Heart Journal, November 1, 2001.

With this type of neuroimmunologic healing, doesn't it make sense that diabetes, a disease known to be of autoimmune origin, could benefit from similar treatment? I think so. And for sure it's worth exploring on our own. We don't need permission from anybody to do this. We just need interesting books with new ideas, meditation, prayer, new eating ideas, google, and some ingenuity on our part. It's incredibly empowering to think I might be able to heal myself.

If you want to try this, I say *Go for it!* Please don't go off your medication in the meantime however, because it is supporting your health right now. You need as much health in your physical and psychological bank account as possible to go on this journey. Also, find a physician who is willing to work with you. If your doctor discourages your trying new things, he or she may not be a lot of help for you. Any good researcher keeps records, so devise some kind of journal to document what you do and how your blood sugar reacts. Any time you make a change you'll need to do blood sugar checks every hour or two to be sure you're in a safe range or to take action to get back to a safe range. When you make a change, try it for a couple of weeks if possible, so you can get blood sugar patterns that are reliable. Also, if you see something change, write down everything you can think of that is going on as far as stress, illness, food intake, exercise, medication dose and timing, all the things that affect our bodies. That will help you sleuth out what is really happening. If you find something helps you, but you're not sure about it, stop doing it for a week, then try it again. If the change happens again, you are definitely onto something.

Of course there are researchers out there trying to cure diabetes. But I have to tell you there is something very odd to me in believing that researchers, who have never lived one diabetic day in their lives, will be able to cure a disease they are studying in rats and mice, who not surprisingly are somewhat unlike humans, and rats and mice do not develop diabetes naturally, but have been altered in some way to get the disease. An endocrinologist who is a friend of mine said, "Sure, we know about a hundred ways to cure rats of diabetes, but so far it doesn't work in humans." Well, there you go.

In western medicine there is a huge divide only slightly smaller than the Royal Gorge, between mind and body. Do you know why? If you think it's because that makes sense, you are wrong. Here's the story. In the 1700s Rene DeCartes, the founding father of Cartesian medicine which is practiced in the western hemisphere, wanted to study cadavers to learn more about the human body. He felt he could help his patients better if he knew more about how our insides work. He asked the Pope for permission to dig up dead bodies for his study. It seems odd to me that the Pope was in charge of dead bodies, but regardless, the Pope was very clear in responding with a loud and clear, "No".

Being a determined man, Dr. DeCartes persisted in his requests, and finally the Pope relinquished with one absolute dictate...DeCartes could exhume and study cadavers if, and *only* if, he accepted that medicine had jurisdiction over only the physical body, whereas the church retained complete ownership of the emotional, psychological and spiritual aspects of humanity.

DeCartes accepted the terms, and those of us receiving western medicine have suffered from this schizophrenic split ever since. Wow. It's encouraging to see that the split is narrowing a bit, and our minds and bodies get to make friends with each other more often these days.

There are so many things I would love to tell you, but honestly, I need to get this book to my publisher or you'll never even get to read what I've already written. Let me end with a wonderful story about freedom that I came across in Mother Jones magazine, the January/February 2004 issue, written by Adam Hochschild, and entitled *Against All Odds*. As you read the story, think about diabetes.

In 1787, three-quarters of the population of our entire globe were enslaved, either bought and sold on the slave market, working as indentured servants or bound in serfdom under kings. To imagine a world without slavery at that time, would be as strange as it would be for us to imagine a world without asphalt. On August 1, 1787, the paradigm of slavery began to change.

Olaudah Equiano, a young African man living in England, who had bought his way out of slavery, read a newspaper account that sickened and horrified him. A ship filled with some four hundred-forty enslaved Africans was traveling from Africa to Jamaica, and fell on hard times. The journey was delayed, and during that time water and food became short. Those suffering the worst were slaves held in the hold where they had no fresh air, no system for sanitation, and no fresh water, let alone food. Slaves began dying in droves.

The ship's captain was concerned, as one might imagine, but sadly not because of loss of human life. His concern was that a sick or dead slave would bring him no money at market. He did remember however, that for each slave dying from "natural causes" such as drowning, the captain would receive insurance reimbursement of thirty British pounds in silver. He began having slaves thrown over the side. In all, one hundred thirty-three slaves were "jettisoned". The latter groups began to realize what was being done, and tried to fight for their lives. Because of their resistance, the captain had them bound and gagged before they were thrown over the side. They hadn't even the remotest chance for survival.

When Equiano read the article he was devastated. He began to create anti-slavery pamphlets and letters which he feverishly distributed thoughout Britian. Ultimately this anti-slavery sentiment reached a clergyman named Thomas Clarkson, who vigilantly joined the siege. Equiano assembled a group of twelve men who vowed to *end slavery in their lifetime.*

Fifty-one years later, on August 1, 1837, Emancipation came to the British Empire, the largest empire known to the world at that time. Thomas Clarkson lived to witness his long-desired hope.

Margaret Mead said, "Never doubt that a small group of thoughtful, committed citizens can change the world. Indeed, it is the only thing that ever has."

Can we abolish diabetes from the face of this planet in our lifetimes? Yes. *Absolutely, yes.*

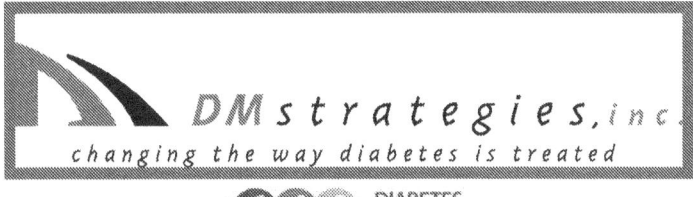

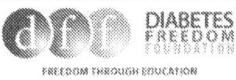

The Diabetes Freedom Foundation (DFF)

Founded in Kansas City in 2004 through contributions from DM Strategies, Inc., the Diabetes Freedom Foundation is a not for profit organization whose mission is *freeing the world from the tyranny of diabetes through education*. DFF and DM Strategies provide and facilitate diabetes education through national training symposia for healthcare professionals, focusing on endocrinologists, endocrine fellows, primary care physicians and residents, and other specialists who interact with diabetic patients and their families. Within Kansas City, DFF provides diabetes education for those who have the disease or want to know more about it.

Examples of programs include:

- **Diabetes Training Forums** – programs are held in collaboration with DM Strategies, Inc. and the Endocrine Fellows Foundation. Forums provide education regarding the most up to date standards of care, and using a team approach to diabetes.
- **Diabetes and Cardiovascular Disease** - more than 750 attendees participated in these seminars. The CME program, accredited for 4 hours, was held in locations across the United States, for endocrinologists, cardiologists, and primary care physicians.
- **Diabetes Enduring Materials** – CME accredited programs regarding diabetes and cardiovascular disease risk-assessment, prevention and treatment, have been provided to physicians who opt in, across the United States.
- **Public Education** – local Kansas Citians receive public education through seminars on diabetes. More than 300 healthcare professionals and lay attendees participated in the first annual seminar held November 11, 2006, at the Overland Park Convention Center. The program offers a

half-day of didactic lectures, followed by an afternoon of workshops, hands-on use of diabetes equipment, and health screen examinations.

• **Education Grants** – Diabetes Exercise Imperium was funded in 2006 at Kansas University Medical Center - Department of Physical Therapy. The program offers ongoing instruction in exercise methods, specific to each diabetic person's need and level. Exercise practice is increased slowly over time, so each user ultimately understands his/her capacity, and graduates to continue independent exercise.

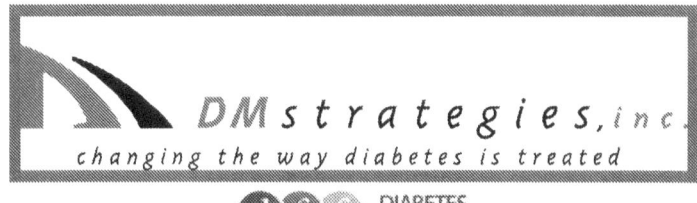

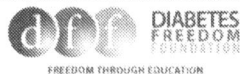

NATIONAL ADVISORY COMMITTEE

The National Advisory Committee for DM Strategies, Inc. and Diabetes Freedom Foundation meets annually to facilitate discovery and evaluation of diabetes national trends, studies, drug releases, research, and provocative thinking relevant for healthcare professionals in diabetes. This wealth of information underpins the most compelling needs facing the care, treatment and prevention of diabetes today.

Members of the advisory panel include Endocrinologists, Primary Care Physicians, Cardiologists, Diabetes Nurse Educators, Nutritional Specialists, Behavioral Psychologists, and Basic Researchers in Diabetes.

2006 – 2010 National Advisory Committee Members

- Andrew Drexler, MD, Professor of Medicine UCLA, Los Angeles, CA
- Vivian Fonseca, MD, Tulane University, New Orleans, LA
- Royce Keilers, DO, American Diabetes Association Primary Care Liaison, Austin, TX
- Steven Marso, MD, Mid-America Heart Institute, Kansas City, MO
- Charles A. Reasner, MD, Texas Diabetes Institute UTHSCSA, San Antonio, TX
- David C. Robbins, MD, Diabetes Institute KUMC, Kansas City, KS
- Lisa Stehno-Bittel, PhD, Diabetes Institute KUMC, Kansas City, KS

- William H. Polonsky, PhD, CDE, Behavioral Diabetes Institute, San Diego, CA
- Richard R. Rubin, PhD, CDE, Johns Hopkins, Baltimore, MD
- Belinda P. Childs, RN, MSN, ARNP, CDE, Mid-America Diabetes Associates, Wichita, KS
- Ruth Mencl, RN, MN, CDE, St. Luke's Diabetes Center, Kansas City, MO
- Marion J. Franz, RD, LD, CDE, Nutrition Concepts by Franz Inc., Minneapolis, MN
- Diane Reader, RD, LD, CDE, International Diabetes Center, Minneapolis, MN

Table 1 - Insulins

Brand Name	Generic Name	Manufacturer	Onset of Action	Peak Action (hours)	Duration of Action (hours)
RAPID ACTING					
Apidra®	insulin glulisine	Sanofi-Aventis	< 15 min.	1 - 2	3 - 4
Humalog®	insulin lispro	Eli Lilly and Company	< 15 min.	1 - 2	3 - 4
Novolog®	insulin aspart	Novo Nordisk, Inc.	< 15 min.	1 - 2	3 - 4
REGULAR					
Humulin R®	regular	Eli Lilly and Company	0.5 – 1 hour	2 - 3	3 - 6
Novolin R ReliOn® (Wal-Mart)	regular	Novo Nordisk, Inc.	0.5 – 1 hour	2 - 3	3 - 6
INTERMEDIATE ACTING					
Humulin N®	NPH lispro protamine	Eli Lilly and Company	2 – 4 hours	4 – 10	10 - 16
Novolin N® ReliOn (Wal-Mart)	NPH	Novo Nordisk, Inc.	2 – 4 hours	4 – 10	10 - 16
LONG ACTING					
Levemir®	insulin detemir	Novo Nordisk, Inc	0.8 – 2 hours	minimal peak	up to 24
Lantus®	insulin glargine	Sanofi-Aventis	2 – 4 hours	mostly peakless	20 - 24

Brand Name	Generic Name	Manufacturer	Onset/Peak/Duration
MIXTURES			
Humalog Mix 50/50®	50% lispro protamine 50% insulin lispro	Eli Lilly and Company	Combination
Humulin 70/30®	70% NPH 30% regular	Eli Lilly and Company	Combination
Novolin 70/30® ReliOn® (Wal-Mart)	70% NPH 30% regular	Eli Lilly and Company	Combination
NovoLog Mix 70/30®	70% aspart protamine 30% aspart	Novo Nordisk, Inc.	Combination

Adapted from Diabetes Forecast, *Resource Guide 2007*: page RG15